THE SORCERER'S APPRENTICE

THE
SORCERER'S
APPRENTICE

TALES OF THE MODERN HOSPITAL

SALLIE TISDALE

McGRAW-HILL BOOK COMPANY
New York • St. Louis • San Francisco
Hamburg • Mexico • Toronto

The author and publisher gratefully acknowledge permission to reproduce previously published material: From "Fire and Ice" in *The Poetry of Robert Frost* edited by Edward Connery Lathem. Copyright 1923, © 1969 by Holt, Rinehart and Winston. Copyright 1951 by Robert Frost. Reprinted by permission of Holt, Rinehart and Winston, Publishers. From *Waiting for God* by Simone Weil, translated by Emma Craufurd, copyright 1951 by Simone Weil, by permission of the Putnam Publishing Group. From *A Fortunate Man* by John Berger, copyright John Berger by permission of Pantheon Books, a Division of Random House, Inc. From *A Grief Observed* by C. S. Lewis, © 1961 N. W. Clerk. Published by Winston Seabury Press, Minneapolis, Minnesota. All rights reserved. Used with permission. From *The Inferno* by Dante Alghieri, translated by John Ciardi. Copyright © 1954, 1982 by John Ciardi. Reprinted by arrangement with New American Library, New York, New York. From *Psychoanalysis of Fire* by Gaston Bachelard, by permission of Beacon Press. From *Emotional Care of the Facially Burned and Disfigured* by Norman Bernstein, by permission of Little, Brown & Co. From *Awakenings* by Oliver Sacks, by permission of Duckworth. From "The Abyss" by Theodore Roethke, by permission of Doubleday. Portions of Chapter 11 first appeared in *Co-Evolution Quarterly* #41.

1 2 3 4 5 6 7 8 9   FGR FGR   8 7 6

ISBN 0-07-064784-4

LIBRARY OF CONGRESS CATALOGING-IN-PUBLICATION DATA

Tisdale, Sallie.
  The sorcerer's apprentice.
  1. Hospital patients—Psychology. 2. Hospitals—
Psychological aspects. 3. Medical ethics. I. Title.
RA965.3.T57 1986   174'.2   85-23961
ISBN 0-07-064784-4

Book design by Mary A. Wirth

To my children

ACKNOWLEDGMENTS

The following institutions graciously assisted me: Holladay Park Hospital, Emanuel Hospital, Providence Medical Center, the Oregon Health Sciences University, all in Portland, Oregon; Harborview Medical Center in Seattle; Pacific Medical Center and Mt. Zion Hospital and Medical Center in San Francisco; U. C. Davis Medical Center in Sacramento, California; and the Oregon Regional Primate Research Center in Beaverton, Oregon.

Thanks to Jim England, R.N., Kathie Mallory, R.N., Carolyn Dare, R.N., Mary McBride, R.N., Rosalyn Harper, R.N., Virginia O'Leary, R.N., Beverly Webber, R.N., Arlene Austinson, R.N., Ruth Barstow, R.N., Paul Bailey, M.D., Richard Zimmerman, M.D., Harold Spies, M.D., and Nancy Alexander, M.D.

My personal thanks to my agent, Katinka Matson, my assistant, Lori Cauthorn Lakey, Laura Dolan, who helped with typing, and my editor, Tom Miller, as well as many encouraging friends. Thank you, Bill, for your trenchant comments.

I am especially grateful to the many nurses who took me in as one of their own, and treated me with willingness and understanding. I am proud to be a member of that clan, and sorry so many must remain nameless. All the stories, characters, and conversations that follow are true and unpolished. To protect the privacy of many and the confidence of those who shared their secrets, I have used pseudonyms throughout.

Finally, I remember Chuck Ryberg, who has certainly forgotten me, and that many years ago he made me write when I thought there might be better things to do.

Sallie Tisdale

Contents

Far-Flung Machines and Tinkering

O LIVE WAS KNOWN AS A DIFFICULT PATIENT, A COM-
plainer. She suffered an enormous wound in her
back from complications after the removal of a cancerous
lung. The elaborate dressing changes had been done twice
a day for several months and promised to continue for
months more. After the first weeks Olive had developed
the disconcerting habit of telling her nurses how to do
the job, which packages to open in what order, how to
lay the materials out across the table. She was as attentive
and critical as our teachers in nursing school. When Olive
got upset, she couldn't talk for a moment, and the edges
of the wound would gape open and then close in the
rhythm of her breath. Her words, when they came, whis-
tled hoarsely; I had to wait for a pause before I could
stuff more gauze past the lips of the hole.

She was difficult to care for, bearing such a grave insult.
One day as I gathered up the trash off her bed she caught

my eye and smiled slightly. "I know it's just a dressing to you," she said, panting for air in the remaining lung. "But to me it's my life."

O LIVE SHOULD HAVE DIED, OF COURSE. "TWENTY, TEN, five years ago, this person—these people—would have died," I am told again and again by professionals proud to point out their accomplishments. Miracles they are, too: medicine has created whole populations that never before existed. It promises more—whole new realms of people. Premature babies so young and unfinished we see in them our relationship to fish, burn victims with faces cloaked in scars, dialysis patients whose blood runs before their eyes—miracles all, all suffering.

In my moments with them lies a secret and illuminating experience. These are moments of harrowing physical pain, undiluted fear, and a kind of relentless grief that grips the heart in a fist. All this is a gift given to people who should have died, who can thank me and my medical peers for their extra time. They clamor for help, for an explanation of this dubious gift; we don't seem to have the will to respond. An odd lethargy grips us, carrying us like a cork on the surf, and we bob along, unprotesting. We can, therefore we do.

They want help, these people. So do I. We need help in coming to terms with the suffering, help in answering certain fundamental questions, help in asking the questions in the first place. This need is far beyond economic handwringing or ethics committees. It demands an acknowledgment of the surreal reality of the sick and of the maelstrom in which health professionals strain for balance.

The sick have always held a special place. They are

granted a temporary annulment of responsibility, a kind of magic, as though they are less rooted to this world. (The sick are freed of certain boundaries of imagination by the constriction of their physical and psychological limits.) The body fails; the mind literally wanders. Despite its magical qualities, this state is desired by no one (though we may often want the annulment it contains), and the sense we have of its special purpose is unconscious, even visceral—as though we feel it in our bodies and not our intellect. What our bodies feel is the proximity of death.

Still there is our powerlessness in the face of immense skill. It is a cognitive dissonance of sorts, as the distance between us, one person to another, increases. This dissonance is due, in part, to the fecundity of the technology, the sheer weight of machinery. We lament, we worry, and yet the surf catches us and sweeps us out to sea. We wave farewell to the shore, never thinking to jump ship and swim back. We've forgotten how to swim.

I WANT TO GET AT THE REASONS FOR THE STRANGE STATE of amnesia we in the health professions find ourselves in. I want to find clues to my weird experiences, try to sense the nature of being sick. Surely in all the stories I see and hear there is a key, a password, a passage.

I am a registered nurse; I have a bachelor's degree in the discipline. In the parlance of the 1980s, this makes me a "professional" nurse. I am versed not only in the bedpan and syringe but also in theories of research, principles of teaching, and techniques of management. I entered nursing school as anyone enters a profession, for a multitude of reasons. Mine included a struggle of many years' duration with a chronic illness. I was mildly disabled by pain for a time, had several hospital stays, endured several surgeries. I lost a part of my body, gave it up to the surgeon and the incinerator. I had long been fascinated by the body, its astonishing intricacy, the labyrinthine twists and improbable turns of physiology. I'd dissected cadavers, worked in nursing homes. And most of all, I wanted to understand what had happened to me and what had been done to me—and from that understand what happens to us all.

I took on the role of the nurse, the image, and promptly left the hospital. Most of my time has been spent in nursing homes, where I feel more comfortable. I like old people; I like seeing them every day, the same faces. I like being around mostly nurses, and not so many medical students, technicians, administrators, and insurance review artists. I like being able to work on a problem for a while, chew over it, try this and that, before people are snatched from my hands. I try to stay on my technical toes by working the occasional shift in a local hospital, but hospitals make me nervous. To me the hospital is an odd place, a difficult place, most of all, a hard place to be sick.

When I first tried my hand at nursing, I was rough and fearful. I assumed that with time and experience I would acquire the smoothness of the expert. This was the promise—that it would someday be natural—and it is. The shaky hands are long gone. I have acquired a grace of sorts. I can work with one eye on the clock, a negligence toward my routine chores that is the stuff of professionals.

But one set of skills has led to a new kind of ignorance. Alongside familiarity crouches caution and doubt, and I don't think improving my hand-eye coordination or reading another textbook is going to help. At times nursing seems a strange discipline, requiring of me unnatural behavior, because being sick is the strangest of states and is most unnatural. Some days the hair on the back of my neck stands up, as though a breeze had blown very quietly by.

I began by wanting to understand how my body worked. Now, that isn't enough. The illness and pain I witness have a hallucinatory quality to them. There is suspense in them, and suspension: I float with my patients in a place set aside especially for us. The physical pain—tumor pressing on nerve, swollen, arthritic joints—doesn't worry me much. Often I would like to take away this gnawing, hungry pain, but I don't despair in its presence. But—and this is where it all turns, where I spin on my toes out of balance—I see more. I see what we've created with our headlong, hard-pressed, slapdash sprint for perfection. I need to explain not just my body, not just my job—I need to explain myself to myself.

Part of the mystery is simply the mystery of illness. Being sick is unnatural. Erosion, obviously, is natural. Our physical bodies are essentially entropic. What I speak of is the series of discretely framed moments that make up the day of the sick, the changed perception, the changed priorities, when a glass of water can take on enormous meaning and value.

Another part of the mystery is what I do about that glass of water. Caring for the sick is a queer way to spend one's time, and we act as though it were the most normal thing in the world—as though it were just a job. I prod sensitive places. I concern myself with the immediate, that small, tense space generated around each bed and held in by a thin yellow curtain. My patients (they *are* mine; I own the time I spend with them) have concerns of their own. I am a violator, a trespasser, a Peeping Tom. And I am also privileged (if I choose) to hand out little mercies along the way, a tip of the cap and some figurative silver on their palms. Do I stop my momentum, reverse, go get the drink of water? It depends.

I am struck now by how little we recognize the eccentricity of this relationship. How can we forget the fine line that separates us? The malfunctions of the human body are so illogical and bizarre that at times they seem a frightening joke—a practical joke where the humor (like all good humor) lies in an unexpected juxtapositioning and the element of surprise. And we're always surprised.

Quivering like jelly, hiding under the covers, we are sought out by the treachery of decay. We are given a gift-wrapped pain all our own, unbidden, with a variety of faces. Here is your tumor (and perhaps mine): a Cheshire cat, swollen and sure. Attacked by the poison of chemotherapy, the thing seems to disappear, leaving only a sly and superior grin, a reminder of its presence, of where it sat a moment ago. You cannot shake the memory, and you cannot shake the sensation either, the heaviness and weighing down.

People who are sick and pained are in a state of surrender. Its quality exists outside category, outside and beyond such details as diagnosis and prognosis. Patients yield to this condition whether or not they want to, whether or not they are aware of doing so. A gallbladder removed, a broken leg, cancer—each person with such a loss renders up an external identity. One is no longer a mother or daughter or wife. One is not a banker or plumber, a gardener or tennis player. Nothing holds; the self acquiesces. One becomes a patient, a body—wholly a body—so that the dissection can begin.

Here is examination without regard for borders, without consideration for the brittle delicacies underneath. You must describe the details, find words for the wordless. Things happen to you and you don't know their names. You are not expected to understand, only to submit. "Now," says the examiner, knife in hand, "let us see what is inside." He means to find that which has been hidden. We in the business call patients like Olive—trying to hold onto themselves in spite of the onslaught, daring to remind us that one loss needn't lead to others—difficult. They have not accomplished—not yet—a successful adjustment to the sick role.

H OW HAVE WE COME TO SUCH A PASS? MUST WE SPIN out of control, meeting pain with pain, grief with grief, death with a prolonged dying? We should not be wholly unfamiliar with the place in which we find ourselves. The industrial revolution skewed our social relations; our ability to act grew faster than our ability to comprehend the meaning of our actions. A disruption of the same kind is the dissonance in medicine—water lapping at the toes of the sorcerer's apprentice, who wanted the power but couldn't grasp the consequences.

Medicine, based in science, is linear. A set of symptoms leads to a diagnosis, which leads to treatment, which leads to side effects, remission, a change. Linear thinking always creates a kind of linear intent, and there's the trick. What exactly are we trying to accomplish? Might this disruption be partly because the patient wants something different from what the doctor wants—in fact, something that isn't linear at all?

Oliver Sacks is a neurologist who came to understand this in his work with people who suffered from severe Parkinson's disease, people whose symptoms had so bound them that their surrender was nearly total—as Sacks puts it, the disease was "infinite." He writes of our unspoken, inarticulate feeling of loss—we who were once whole are now shattered—and of the way in which this metaphysical belief is twisted by medical authorities. The sick person desires a grand change, a lifting of the veil, and the doctor offers *things*—pills, treatments, procedures. "Health, thus conceived," writes Sacks, "is reduced to a *level*, something to be titrated or topped-up in a mechanical way." Thus do we differentiate—thus does the euclidean purpose of the practitioners cause a greater distance, a darker veil.

I see it in doctors' aggression. I see it in their walks, as they stride through the wards, swinging stethoscopes in an arc broad enough to define the space they mean to claim. I see how tough even young doctors are, or try to be. And research strides on too in big and booming steps.

Researchers mean to find the truth of a story, fit a piece into the puzzle—the flat puzzle, the reproduction that lies on the table—however small. They may know it all! Like gamblers who have stayed too long at the table, unwilling to leave until the pot is divided, these are the purveyors of new miracles, huddled around a table in a dark room, beneath a swaying light bulb. Who will quit first, cut his losses, go home? Who will risk the derision of his fellows? The uncertainty grows; new skills bring new questions. But don't ask. Any notice of the irony involved brings only a territorial defensiveness, lest we seek for deeper meanings, lest we look, not just at means, but at ends. (After an infant girl nicknamed Baby Fae received a transplanted baboon heart a physician said, "Objections to the procedure will undoubtedly be lodged on a variety of grounds, some of which will be emotional rather than clearly rational.") When the weapon is more powerful than its wielder, a show of bravado seems in order. Meanwhile, a patient lies on the table, waiting, worried. I must do something.

All these miracles, the achievements of this flexed-muscle medicine, do more: they push *me* away, sidle between me and the patient. My value, my entire purpose, changes. Am I care giver or clinical specialist, servant or professional?

Listen to a doctor who wants to put robots in hospitals

and nursing homes: "We don't want to depersonalize nursing homes, but many nursing tasks are boring, difficult, unpleasant, and demeaning for both patient and caretaker." Tasks like "toileting, bathing, feeding, transferring, and grooming." Where am I? I am down the hall, monitoring the robots on a closed-circuit screen while I have a cup of coffee. The patient, taken firmly in a steel hand, is presumed pleased.

Perhaps the most closely guarded secret in the hospital is the pity of the healthy for the sick. We are contemptuous of them. The bad jokes, the slang, the name-calling are passed off as a tension release. Often they are. But we also feel a superiority, in part because we claim to understand the mysteries. We are the perpetrators of the mysteries. We can neither face our own decay nor live with what we do to others—to our fellows, our twins. Sick people are different, alien; they have allowed this thing to happen to them. That's why health professionals make the worst patients, the most irascible and demanding. The sick are expatriate, weak—fish out of water flopping embarrassingly on the sidewalk.

Ask a physician, nurse, medical researcher, or bioengineer why he or she is in that line of work and you'll very likely get one of several answers: because it's interesting, because it's challenging or stimulating, because the money's good. A lot of people will say they would like, in whatever small way they can, to ease some of the pain in this sad world that surrounds us.

This last is a noble sentiment and, I think, almost always sincere. I share it. Taped to my refrigerator is a cartoon of two middle-aged and overweight men dressed in suits and ties. One says to the other: "I used to ask myself, 'What can I do to help my fellow man?' But I couldn't think of anything that wouldn't have put me to considerable inconvenience." I suspect that easing the suffering of others is always inconvenient. To do so, one must stop deflecting the pain, stop the evasion, take the nose up from the ground. The fact remains that much—not a little—of modern medical treatment is painful and damaging in and of itself and that as this pain increases, so does our sense of powerlessness.

Yes, I know about serendipity, victorious cures, and heroics and second chances. How we have built ourselves up! And how we demand compensation for our troubles. We are restless and can't name the cause. We wash the faces of people hanging by their toes over death and think of . . . something else.

WHAT TO DO, WHAT TO DO, WHERE TO BEGIN? LET US begin at the beginning. Let us look at one another. John Berger speaks of recognition, of what it means for one person to know another. Recognition, he explains, is nothing more than "the truth about a man." In his book about an English country doctor named Sassall, he tells us: "Once he was putting a syringe deep into a man's chest. There was little question of pain but it made the man feel bad: the man tried to explain his revulsion: 'That's where I live, where you're putting the needle in.' 'I know,' Sassall said, 'I know what it feels like. I can't bear anything done near my eyes, I can't bear to be touched there. I think that's where I live, just under and behind my eyes.'" This revelation is what makes Sassall a good doctor, a doctor who can assuage the pain of his patients. He admits his likeness to them, admits his fear. Much of what we do admits nothing of the kind; in fact it has taken the places where we live and sealed them off, locked the door. Elaine Scarry describes her full-length treatise on the experience of pain as being "about the way other persons become visible to us, or cease to be visible to us."

Without prompting, a young dialysis patient points out to me the plastic tube permanently sewn into her forearm, the curve that rears up under the skin: "This is my life, sticking out here." What has she been given, this girl? She is married to a machine.

When all is said and done, though, she doesn't mind her tube. Not really: she is alive in an age of science, she is surrounded by competent, well-meaning people, and a few years ago she would have died. But I tell you it is strange.

Recognition requires us to heed our losses. It is harder when we mask our faces, fail to look like—or at—ourselves. We've even forgotten what we fear, what raises the hair on the backs of our necks. All these dilemmas are incommodious.

This embarrassed duality, if you will, is what so colors the wretched public wringing of hands in the name of medical ethics. It is also why a surgeon finds nothing odd in comparing artificial heart recipients to games in a baseball series. Medical ethics as a concept is doomed to futility. It is too small to contain the problem it hopes to solve. Ethics is the study of conduct and behavior, the study of response, antiphony, echo. Ethics is inherently fluid—fluid, as in provisional. It is the reaction of last resort, the thumb in a dike. Given a certain situation, given A and B in this relation, what should we do? How should we respond? Yet A and B rarely fall into the imagined relation, as one had hoped, and when they do we find that our imagined reply hasn't the gratifying power of conclusion we had hoped it would have. Things linger, slip out, slip away. This kind of ethics is simply more linear intent. It is cerebral, and those who hope to find more than temporary guidance in it are kidding themselves. Relying on medical ethics to spare us difficult decisions is to run ahead of the wave after the dike breaks.

Thus far, we haven't thought deeply enough about our

creations. We haven't *felt* deeply enough; we agonize by committee. We trail behind our far-flung machines and tinkering, using ethics like a map to get from one place on a line to another. It's time to stop and wonder: what are we doing here? Where do we want to go? Having set off smartly in one direction, isn't it possible we'd rather take another trip?

What else? Morality. To many, morality implies cloudy thinking, intuition, a kind of rigid irrationality. A bad word, in these enlightened times of science and linear intent. Morality is the study not of conduct but of purpose. Moral philosophies seek not to be the response but the motivation for the response—for infinite responses, infinite courses rising from a center, meeting infinite puzzles.

John Paris, a theologian, says that "the elevation of technology to the ultimate value" has taken us "far from the kind of wisdom every caring grandmother would know how to apply to these questions." He is on to something. He knows the wind is high, that it blows whispers of religion, instinct, seeking. Something whispers in our hearts, teases at the edge of mere knowledge, mumbles to us if we would just shut up and listen.

More than one person has tried to stretch medical ethics into a kind of medical morality. Theologians usually make the noble attempt. But as ethics is too small, so is medicine. The moral inadequacy that has allowed us, like lemmings, to run together blindly is greater than medicine. It encompasses in its impotence more than the relatively simple life-and-death decisions that ethics committees are called on to make. We're all in this together—we're all getting old, and sick, and dying. We need a morality of sickness and health—of helplessness and power, difference and sameness, compassion and pain.

I have stood by the bed of a brain-damaged man, a man whose brain had burst with blood and been sucked into his spine like a sausage crammed into its casing, stood there watching his lungs fill up with air and deflate only because of the respirator next to his bed, heard his heart beat only because of the drugs dripping into his veins. I was just a student nurse. I stood at the back, behind the physicians who couldn't decide what to do, who seemed not to know what to do even as they knew what had to be done.

What makes the difference, that I didn't share that indecision? I would have flipped the switch, pulled the plug, hopped a train for home without a backward glance, without an apology. Left alone with him, I bent over his ear and apologized for not doing just that. Am I more—or as some would have it, less—humane than the physicians? Does my comparative lack of biochemical knowledge render me somehow blissfully ignorant—or knowledgeable of other things? Perhaps I am simply more willing to live with death, less willing to live with and accept unnatural pain. If so, it is because of my intent, my purpose, and that's where we can begin to search. I suspect there's more.

Children expect hardship, expect the world to be out of control. Certainly they tell us about it: they scream and cringe and clutch the siderails, tear up the sheets and throw the rice pudding on the floor. Sick, they cry out for mother—but grown men are not permitted to cry in homesickness from their hospital beds, and neither are the doctors and nurses who care for them. This is loneliness exquisite. If we are in this together, then we are in it as children, as innocents, wondering what's been lost.

In a very important sense, the sick have no voice. If they did they might not know the words; in fact, there might not *be* words, singular and telling, for what is happening here. No reductionism, no definition, can embrace it.

And this, then, is what I mean to do. Every morality

has its moral tales, vignettes that illuminate and, perhaps, explain. These stories are parables, fables, of brave, lonely people powerful in their helplessness, surrounded by machines. Those big, blinking things hovering over us— what are they for but to delineate us one from the other, refine the limits? Here, this skin and vessel, this is your boundary. It is as close to you as I can get, it is all I can see. We have extended ourselves and our measurements. We see and hear beyond our given range, probe bloodlessly in the dark interiors, congratulate ourselves on progress. But when the beam comes sliding over and it's *us* underneath—you, me, suddenly a fish out of water— we're speechless. It is as though we don't know anything after all.

FASTER THAN A CHEETAH AT SPRINT

A ARON, FIVE YEARS OLD, AT FIRST HAD SUFFERED A HEAD-ache and a sore throat. Just a summer cold, perhaps a slight flu. After a few days, the symptoms still stubbornly refused to improve. His mother, Leah, confined him to bed and kept a close eye. Just a tenacious virus, she thought, until the third afternoon.

Leah peeked in on Aaron, where she had left him look-ing at picture books, and found him slack and quiescent. His faint answers were insensible, confused. The borders had shifted. How quickly things change. Leah felt a tingle on the back of her neck, a bit lost. Suddenly this was no summer cold.

Leah spent a few moments calling neighbors, her hus-band, the doctor—making arrangements. She stood in the hall, trailing the long phone cord across the house to watch Aaron while she talked. He lay semiconscious. His forehead was hot and damp; he moved sluggishly away from her hand as though it hurt him to be cradled.

As she reached under him—she herself barely 5 feet tall, thin, stringy, with bottle-bottom glasses that magnified her frightened eyes—to pick him up and carry him to a waiting car, he began to convulse. His whole body became suddenly stiff and resistant, his head flung back; rhythmically, his arms and legs and the muscles of his face began to shake, mechanically, uncontrollably. She stood there and stared at this foreign thing that was her son. When his galloping subsided, she snatched him up, and ran, his head heavy like a stone on her shoulder.

A neighbor drove them to the hospital; Leah sat in the back seat with Aaron's head in her lap. The car turned a corner and he convulsed again, beating a patter against her leg. He had not relaxed before the spasms returned; seizure followed seizure. How dark the sky seemed. Leah stumbled to the door of the emergency room with her awkward, trembling burden. Even as she turned, a wild fear, an incredible prophecy, was forming in her heart.

I F YOU CUT YOUR FINGER ON A DIRTY TIN CAN, YOUR finger may become infected. Bacteria know a deal when they see one and are quick to establish cheap quarters wherever available. Your body immediately sets to work to root it out. The finger swells, the cut becomes warm and red and exquisitely tender. Blood flow is diverted to the wound, along with a fraction of the blood elements designed to kill bacteria. With a little time and relative good health, the cut heals. The pus, made of dead bacteria and wasted antibodies and tissue fluid, drains off, and the skin grows rapidly over. Perhaps not even a small scar will remain.

The system of infection and inflammation fighting over territory works wonders most of the time. The process is uncomfortable for the host, sometimes worse; high fevers are only one of the extremes to which the body will go. In truth, the healthy body's forces attack an infection with a savagery usually associated with barbarian armies. The gloriously heroic sacrifices, the very ostentatiousness, of the immune system are the source of misery and even death. In the wrong place, uncontrolled, the dash forward of inflammation wins only a Pyrrhic victory. Meningitis is one such case.

The central nervous system—the brain and spinal cord—is covered with a tough, three-layered membrane called the meninges. Over and past the membranes, around and behind the cord, and into the brain's central foyer runs a complex closed system of cerebrospinal fluid which serves as the brain's shock absorber. With meningitis, this thin, clear liquid clouds and thickens; the irritation produces the classic—although by no means universal— symptoms: headache and stiff neck.

So many different organisms can be responsible: the *Hemophilus influenzae* bacterium or its pals *Neisseria meningitidis* and *Streptococcus pneumoniae*, also viruses, amoebas, the tuberculosis organism, and the normally benign intestinal bug *Escherichia coli*. These invaders can glide in on the bloodstream after a cold or ear infection. They can wiggle through the hairline crack in the skull after a blow to the head. The amoeba *Naegleria* lives in freshwater lakes and ponds and slips through the nasal membranes of unsuspecting swimmers. Interlopers slide up through a sinus or sneak into a baby's circulation as he glides out his mother's vagina. The meningitis organisms are virulent opportunists, gleeful at finding themselves in such a protein-rich hothouse. But only the weaker hosts succumb.

The intensity of the disease depends a great deal on

the type of organism and the age of the victim. The disease can move faster than a cheetah at sprint, too fast for any human to catch and wrestle to the ground. A few decades ago meningitis killed just about everyone who caught it, and quickly; the infection raced through entire populations. Now the mortality rate is a single-digit number; people recover, given proper treatment, in time.

I N THE EMERGENCY ROOM LEAH WAS SHUT OUT BY THE converging backs that surrounded the child. An IV was inserted, a big needle dripping Valium to stop the seizures. A nurse spoke briefly to her, peering around a curtain—perfunctory questions, what and how long, to establish a history, a reason. The boy was turned on his side and curled up like a fetus, unprotesting, and his back was punctured by a needle as long, it seemed to his mother, as her arm. The needle slid into the thin, tight places between the vertebrae and withdrew a few small spoonfuls of the sap inside. But before the sample of cerebrospinal fluid could be labeled and taken to a lab, Aaron's heart stopped.

The controlled speed increased a notch, the same motions and phrases spit out at a higher frequency, the same uncanny precision of one arm reaching under another without warning, only faster. With a sharp electric shock, Aaron's body was lifted off the bed. Leah stood transfixed; prayers chewed between her teeth. What is happening? The neighbor stood a few feet away, back turned, speechless. Leah closed her eyes and thought she was asleep. The big stretcher with the little boy slid quickly by. Leah reached out as though her wrist were attached to it by a string and the string broke, her arm dropped.

The most common and, almost without exception, most deadly form of meningitis is bacterial. *Hemophilus* alone is responsible for 40 percent of the cases. Bacterial meningitis has other names, almost nicknames in the sly, evasive language of medicine: purulent, suppurative—in other words, pus-forming.

The brain becomes swollen with blood and tissue fluid, its entire surface layered with pus. The pressure in the skull increases until the winding convolutions of the brain are flattened out; the labyrinths straighten, and the heaving hill-and-dale surface is crushed. The infection spreads rapidly to the ventricles of the brain and from there down the spinal cord. Thick, sticky pus forms tiny films of scar tissue that block small passages and stop up the cerebrospinal flow even further. Small veins are blocked, too, and tiny strokes occur all across the brain. Abscesses form, secret pockets of pus. The spreading infection and pressure from the growing turbulent ocean sitting on top of the brain cause permanent weakness and paralysis, blindness, deafness. People who have survived severe cases of meningitis have been left with personality changes, poor memory, impulsive behavior, and retardation.

This soup in the skull causes such damage by leaning on the fragile structures hidden in its lacy reaches. The posterior lobes of the pituitary gland release a hormone called antidiuretic hormone, or ADH. This substance controls part of the complex fluid balance of the body. Damage to the brain can cause a flood of ADH to be excreted. Cells hold on to their water. The excess is pushed into the tissues of the legs, arms, abdomen, face—until the whole body swells like a water balloon, soft, mushy, so that when you poke gently with a finger the dent lingers, white and grotesque.

Meningococcal infections also create a petechial rash, the bursting of tiny capillaries. Tiny red pinpricks, bright and angry, appear on the skin, as well as in the eyes, ears, and lungs. The joints fill with blood and become sore and hot. So many odd complications.

Unchecked, both the infection and the subsequent inflammation blaze through the body like tinder fire. Disrupted and torn by the toxins and pressures, the brain's electrical activity goes haywire, and the messages get garbled. The person becomes first drowsy, then confused, and then flails in seizure to the lightning dance inside. The adrenal glands that squat on top of the kidneys—those tiny dynamos that can make us pant or sweat in fear and rage—suddenly burst with blood, hemorrhaging. The body falls into shock. Without the stimulating secretions of the adrenals, the blood pressure plummets and the veins collapse. Cells begin to die, oxygen-starved, brain and kidney, muscle and heart—then the heart stops.

There is only one cure in traditional medicine, and that is antibiotics. A physician will usually begin a strong broad-spectrum drug as soon as meningitis is suspected and a sample of fluid is drawn. No drug in the world can control, let alone reverse, the headlong fling of infection and inflammation once it reaches a certain point. The antibiotics used—back-alley, street-fighting drugs—can cause deafness, kidney damage, bleeding stomachs. They are all brawn and no brain.

I CAME TO WORK EARLY ONE MORNING, STOPPING AT THE room where one of my patients from the previous day had been. But the door was closed, the nameplate gone. I peeked in and saw Aaron lying in his tangle of tubes, stark faces beside his bed. Peeping Tom again; my own patient was down the hall. The staff moved like undersea divers, slowly, languidly—a death watch.

He couldn't breathe—his brain had forgotten how—so a respirator breathed for him. The big machine rested next to the bed, its slanted front a mess of dials and gauges like a jet cockpit. Above the machine a white bellows rose and fell, rose and fell, as Aaron's lungs expanded and collapsed. The IV in his arm was spiked with norepinephrine, the substance his lost and wasted adrenals could never make again, to keep his heart beating.

Suddenly, a new degree of uncertainty had entered the picture. Without the ventilator, the drugs, the shock in the emergency room, Aaron would have died. Now he is quiescent, half alive. The ability to act, the force at the doctors' fingertips, had pushed Aaron over an edge into a land of limbo, a land where any change would be the result of an active decision, a choice. Without the life support, there would be no choice. Would there be less pain? Which is easier, the blow from heaven or the blow from one's own hand?

The degree of brain damage a person in a coma has suffered can be roughly determined with nothing more than a light, a ballpoint pen, and your fist. First, open the eyes and inspect the dark pupils. Are they wide and staring, are they pinpricks, are the edges smooth or serrated and choppy? Are the eyes equal, or does one seem to envelop the other with its asymmetry? Now shine the light in them, one at a time. Do the pupils contract, or lie inert and vulnerable?

Raise the gown and make a fist, sticking your middle knuckle out sharply. Rub it in the sternum, that sensitive breastbone at the junction of the ribs. Push harder, put your weight behind it. Does the person grunt, try to pull away? Does a hand tense or contract? Now take a fingernail and lay the pen across it. Lean on it, roll it hard across the tender skin, make a bruise. Any reaction? Repeat with a toenail. Now what do you think—as you stand by the bed and call his name softly, does he hear?

But still we must have an electroencephalogram—the EEG—to make the diagnosis. Tiny leads are pierced through the scalp across the whole head to catch and interpret the fearsome flashing inside and translate it into a wandering pattern across a roll of paper. The average conscious person has consistent wave patterns that rise and fall and chatter like the surf. With stimulation—flashing lights, sounds—the waves change in a prescribed and consistent fashion. Deviations, however slight, can mean a great deal to one who reads the language.

If it had been possible to take an EEG of little Aaron as he lay across his mother's lap, the page would have been covered with the Himalayan spikes and valleys of an explosion of electricity. No slow, undulating waves these, but an apocalyptic ion exchange; stilettos, weapons in the Pyrrhic war. Now, however, the boy was still. he did not respond to pain; his eyes stared at the light. An EEG was read carefully and cautiously (for here medicine moves warily) and lay in piles of wide white paper collecting on the floor. The line was flat, unmoving. No spikes here, not even undulations, just a flat line from the pen sliding automatically across the page. We don't trust our eyes or hands or the voice in our heart as much as that pen.

The bellows rose and fell.

Outside the room, at the table where the nurses and residents spread the charts to chat and write, Leah sat. Through the great magnifying glasses her eyes were wet and blank. Next to her sat the social worker, elegantly dressed and calm. Leah stared at me where I huddled over files; the social worker looked at Leah. "Drink this before you go back in," she said, proffering a glass of orange juice. The woman took it and drank, all liquid eyes and angles.

Although the door to Aaron's room remained closed, from the nurse's station one could watch through the windows meant to ease the close supervision such patients require. Aaron had at least one nurse at his bedside all the time; those of us assigned elsewhere able to satisfy our curiosity through glass. We needed to watch. Few details escape the passing conversations of the staff on such a floor—whispers travel. I was a voyeur of another person's nightmare, and the mother knew it.

Another day passed, another EEG. Like a Nebraska highway, the ink flowed. There was nothing left in his skull; it had rotted away, been crushed to pulp, starved, suffocated, and shocked. No antibiotics were going to bring him back now. The respirator puffed gently; a catheter drained off his urine. Perhaps he could have gone on like this for a long while—others have. Eventually his exhausted and dispirited heart would quit again, but hearts can be revived. He had nothing left to worry about, nothing to fear.

A time came in the afternoon of the second day. How these things become told I'll never know; the undersea dance of the staff grew gradually faster. Family gathered in the hall, a united front. Leah and her husband sat by Aaron's bed, and a physician came in to the nurse sitting beside them and gave the orders. He said, "Discontinue the ventilator. Discontinue the IV therapy." Then he duly wrote the words in the progress notes and spun on his heels and left the room.

It was left to the nurse to carry out the orders. She reached up the long transparent tubing of the IV and rolled the clamp closed, stopping the flow. She walked around the bed to the ventilator and flipped a switch. The machine sighed once and stopped.

All was still and hesitant. Then a low wail came rising out of Leah's chest, a lost child's cry, a fetal poem.

———

AARON TRAVELED TO THE MORGUE IN HIS FAVORITE PA-jamas. No matter that in those windowless rooms he'd be undressed before he was cut for the autopsy. Leah had bathed him and combed his hair, straightened his still little limbs. She seemed oblivious to the bright light and the windows. After they were gone, a nurse who'd worked many years in pediatrics told me a story.

"Last year," she said, "we had a two-year-old girl here. She'd fallen down a stairway in her home and broken her neck, high." The nurse wrapped a finger around her throat in illustration. "Her brain stem was damaged; she couldn't breathe. She was gone. We had her on a respirator until the family was ready. But they wanted to donate her kidneys. The person has to be breathing, viable, when the kidneys are removed. So they bundled the little girl into an ambulance, still hooked up, and ran her up to the university where the kidney team is; they took out her kidneys, closed her up, and brought her back here. When she was all settled in bed again and her parents were here, I turned off the machine and she died." The nurse smiled slightly. "I've hardly ever seen a doctor turn off a respirator. They always leave it for the nurses to do."

All over the country I can hear the quiet hum of machines.

BREATHING IN,
BREATHING OUT

I TALK WITH A NURSE WHO BUSIES HERSELF OVER A BADLY burned two-year-old boy who was rescued from a house fire by a fire fighter. "Sometimes the firemen come in to visit the kids, you know, the ones they pulled out—and they wonder if maybe they shouldn't have done it." She looks at the raw, torn skin on the boy's back. The child doesn't clutch the rails, doesn't cry out in homesickness for his mother. His mother died in the fire. He mewls like an animal caught in a trap, bites his pillow, lunges and arches. "I just tell them," finishes the nurse, "that's not for us to decide." This is the riddle. We began it. We beg for more. But we pray to be spared the decisions that must—that always—follow.

Who knows the explanation for the random dice throw that lands one baby here and another safely at home, one child charred and another laughing? We all have our secret theories: we mumble them to ourselves as we care for the losers, because we have to know the reason. How can we bear it if the innocent suffer? How can we explain—to ourselves, to each other—why we must dare the rescue when we despise the result?

Not too long ago sick infants were simply laid to bed and watched—prayed over, perhaps. Nothing could be done; resignation was routine. They depend on us now, utterly, for our good will, but what is not clear is what that good will might entail. With glorious new tools in hand the specialists grant life to even the most hopeless, the most failed, the stumbling leaps of evolution. Now, babies die not from being laid to bed, but from our decision to stop working on them. The birth of a sick or tiny baby, a baby incomplete, puts into motion a gigantic machinery, a humming mammoth of tubes and monitors and scanners that seems to engulf its patrons. The humming is a mantra, an incantation of sorts. We can culture up an egg, stir in a few sperm, but the spell we weave is an abortive one. It's incomplete: once begun, it's out of our hands. How the cells divide, what path they take, and when they emerge to blink at the world is out of our hands.

T HE NEONATAL INTENSIVE CARE UNIT—NICU—IS TUCKED behind closed doors and down a hall. The medical wards opposite have been closed down for lack of patients, and every time I step off the elevator I am struck by the deserted feel. No chance of stumbling on this big, brightly lit room by accident. To get to the tiny patients I have to pass double doors, discouraging signs, obscure machinery, steel carts stacked with linen, and several offices. The people at the desks look up to gaze at me as I pass. Who are you? their expressions ask. Have you the right to be here?

Two floors above is a pediatric unit peopled with older children and teenagers, the near adults. Up there the struggle is not only with illness but also with the beginning glimmers of mortality, the gleam of possible death glimpsed in each other's faces. In NICU and the other nurseries, the plot, the central leitmotiv, is not mortality but pain. Death is not absent, it is just without meaning for patients oblivious to all but the moment: *this* injection, *this* spasm of hunger, *this* bright light and probing hand—moment follows moment, rest follows fitful rest, with little distinction between day and night.

Even the tiniest ones learn the theme, tense when you lean over the crib, their wee hands clenched. Another argument in favor of the nurses' multicolored tops: the babies never come to associate stark white with pain or comfort—they come to expect either—both—from pink and blue and plaid as well. There is no pattern, no definition. We are all enemies and all friends. Diffuse anxiety is in the air like pollen, potent and invisible. Even the plot of pain is obscured by the frailty of the barely born tucked in their sheepskin rugs like sleeping frogs. Because we can't bear to see them born just to die, because of our intent, they come here for a measure of pain, a prescribed suffering, an initiation.

NICU is a room without walls, without curtains to draw round the beds, bright with the overcast sky seen through a bank of windows. A dozen floors up, you often don't see the buildings of the city below, but gaze out across an unbroken overcast. The space is broken up by blocks of machines and chest-high incubators, pillars and sinks and stools, with a long, low desk to one side, crowded with charts and books. Groups of people stand around many of the blocks: nurses with their uniforms covered by hospital gowns, physicians and medical students in brown gowns and green scrubs over suits. They huddle around the bite-size babies stretched out in the cribs, a congregation. Each baby is granted its own nurse; the herd of physicians treats every one, moving from crib to crib as the morning wears on. And again each head comes up, for a moment, to examine me, the newcomer. Are you one of us? Do you belong?

There is no sense of speed, no urgency. We think of "intensive" as meaning a heated rush, all stops out, no holds barred. But all it really means is time. Here the intensity is in the waiting, the vigilance, the time. Knobs are set and drugs chosen; now and then a new drug is added, a setting changed on a machine. For these sick newborns, so early and suddenly plucked from the womb, time will tell.

This particular unit has twenty-three beds, a fairly large number for an NICU. At any one time, 60 to 70 percent of the babies are here because of complications related to their prematurity and the concomitant problems of small size and underdevelopment. The rest of the patients are babies with birth defects or birth injuries and babies awaiting surgery or back from surgery—a few are here with unexplained difficulties. (These last ones are the recipients of a particular moniker. When babies are born without any apparent problem, yet fail to behave, cry, or breathe quite as expected, some doctors refer to them as "FLKs." Without anything to fall back on but their intuition—although many doctors may prefer to call it a trained sense of observation—they feel sure the baby has a problem. The FLK, or Funny-Looking Kid, comes to the nursery to be watched.) But of all these types, it is the premature babies, or "preemies," who exemplify the ward.

I T IS HARD TO DESCRIBE HOW SMALL MOST SUCH BABIES
are. They are a bit longer than a Barbie doll and have
the same heft balanced in your hand as a good-sized package of hamburger. Their heads are too big for their bodies, a peculiarity of fetal growth that will correct itself in
time. For now the heads bob like basketballs balanced on
thin stalks. They lack fat and are bony, emaciated, with
abdomens that swell and distend with feedings. These
weanlings are so light that carrying them gives none of
that satisfactory sense of weight in the arms that comes
from a full-term baby. You have to double-check to be
sure you have them. They are feathers—you pick them
up and they come off the sheet as though gravity had no
hold.

They are also unbearably fragile; in fact, they are rarely
held at all. For the brittle ones, the ones who dance neatly
round a crisis for days or weeks at a time, the slightest
manipulation can disrupt the balance. They are touched
only when necessary: a stroke now and then, the hourly
turn, and what fiddling with tubes and bandages must be
done.

Twenty years ago sick premature babies rarely survived. By five years ago, however, improvements in treatment stretched the boundary past 1 kilogram of weight
—2.2 pounds—and it was then thought to be a magic
number, perhaps the critical number. Yet the borderline
keeps shifting, down to 750 grams, even 500 grams in a
few cases. More and more it is clear that weight matters
less than age and development—what is called gestational
age, age in the womb. A well-developed baby weighing
750 grams will do better than an immature infant weighing half again as much. There is no substitute for the
placenta (although attempts to duplicate it are at hand),
and all the zealousness in the world can't grow a good
lung. For now, the mid-1980s, a baby born two-thirds
through a pregnancy has at least a chance at survival.

Pediatrics and infant care have never been my specialty. I can't claim years of nursing experience or an abiding professional interest. Aaron helped cure me of any innocent notions about saving little children; at the time of his death, my own son was the same age. Whatever we do to adults is more dangerous when it is done to children—whether it is zealous concern, abundant effort, or abandonment of hope. Somehow the power of the sick intensifies when the sick are children who have already surrendered their identities by virtue of their age and innocence. As I visit the NICU, ask technical questions, and rock beside the cribs, a quiet shock passes through me, again and again, like the aftershocks of an earthquake that are felt in the bones, in the passage of messages across the neurons, before they are recognized. It is like a held breath that must be let go. One knows something has happened—a force had made its presence felt—without knowing what or why.

Today the unit holds only nine children for the many beds. Two Isolettes—plastic-enclosed incubators with holes to reach through for handling the baby—hold a pair of twins, boy and girl. The girl weighed only 690 grams at birth. These two, like three others, have respiratory distress syndrome (RDS, also called hyaline membrane disease), the lung affliction that is the penultimate problem of the premature. Between 1968 and 1978, RDS caused 19.5 percent of all infant deaths and was the leading cause of infant mortality in nine of those eleven years.

Little Dale Farwell is one such infant. He weighs a tad under 4 pounds and is four days old, born six weeks early. He rests in an open cradle, waist-high to the adults around him.

In Dale's mouth is a stiff plastic tube that threads into his lungs; it is attached by a hose to a small ventilator tucked behind the rocking chair. The ventilator is forcing him to breathe at a particular rate air that is 25 percent oxygen. He takes breaths of his own as well, in between the set rising and falling of his chest that is governed by the machine.

Into his belly button runs a UA line, an umbilical artery IV that takes advantage of the outsized vessels so recently a part of his umbilical cord. This line is fed by a small glass bottle hung over his head, filled with a mixture of sugar water and salts, with a little heparin added to prevent blood clots from forming in the line. Before the fluid reaches Dale's circulation, it passes through a filter and an automatic pump to ensure its freedom from impurities and bubbles of air and to slow its course to a mere 7 milliliters—about half a tablespoon. Dale has already finished two prescriptions of antibiotics.

On both sides of Dale's chest and on his right thigh are pasted electrodes to measure his heart rate and rhythm, as well as his breathing. Wires lead to a small machine on the shelf over his head, tracing red lines that chase each other across the page. The little racing heart, still tuned to the world in utero, beats 141 quick lub-dubs a minute, then 130, then 167. His breaths are timed, for now, by the ventilator. If his breathing or heartbeat slow or stop, an alarm will sound, a steady unbroken beep.

There is more. On Dale's lower right abdomen, about where his appendix waits under the skin, is another electrode called a transcutaneous oxygen monitor, or TCO_2. It is heated, and it measures the flow of oxygen through his surface tissue circulation. And on Dale's belly is a flat gray button that connects to the bank of heating lights above his bed and signals a change in his temperature. His uncircumcised penis is covered with the plastic lid from a baby bottle to keep him from squirting a urine stream all over his various electrodes.

Dale is lit by an ultraviolet bulb that snakes on a long

arm from the cabinet behind. He is a little jaundiced—that is, his liver is unable to clean the toxic bilirubin, a metabolic by-product, out of his system. Sunshine is the best source of ultraviolet light, but Dale won't be going out to sunbathe. The rays from the bulb help to break down the bilirubin to a safe form.

Dale's nurse Sue measures his blood pressure, temperature, pulse, and respirations every two hours. His urine and blood are tested for sugar every four hours. The amount of oxygen, carbon dioxide, and bicarbonate in his blood (blood gases) is measured every two hours. He is weighed and bathed once a day and turned slightly now and then. His many monitors prevent a face-down posture, so Sue has cut a gauze mask to protect his eyes from the light; it rests on his face like aviator glasses. All this rigmarole, and more to come, is because of his impudence at being born so unexpectedly young.

The stark fact is that premature babies are simply unready to leave the dark surf of the uterus; their organs are unprepared, unfinished, still sculpted in the roughest form. Born so young, they are likely to be covered with fine, silky hair across their faces and down on their limbs. Their skin is sticky with the cheesy vernix that keeps them supple in the womb. They are not ready to eat, not ready to keep themselves warm, not ready to breathe. All these functions must be controlled by the new environment; they have only to lie there getting older, old enough.

The foremost difficulty of premature babies is breathing. Before birth, the fetal lungs are filled with fluid, and the tiny alveoli—little sacs that will expand with air after birth and become the essential component of the lung—are collapsed, turned in upon themselves, dormant. When a fully grown baby is born, after the violent work of labor and the jarring sensory shock of the unfetal world, the lungs expand with a great gasp. Within a few minutes, most of the fluid is absorbed, the alveoli yawning after their long sleep and filling with intoxicating, oxygen-rich air. The blood flow to the lungs increases as much as tenfold. An hour after birth, the expert movement of air in the lungs is like that of a young adult.

Premature babies like Dale can't always manage that first great gasp, partly because they have escaped the stimulating trauma of labor by virtue of their size or birth by cesarean section and partly because, for reasons unknown, their chemistry is somehow deficient. The interior of healthy infant lungs is covered with a lipid material called surfactant, which acts as a detergent. Surfactant reduces surface tension so that liquid slides off the lining and the alveoli can bloom and flower.

No one knows why, but premature babies have insufficient surfactant, which leads to a vicious, potentially lethal cycle. The lungs become stiff, "noncompliant," stubbornly refusing to stretch, so each breath is as difficult as the first one. Premature babies must labor for each breath until they are exhausted, working on increasingly less oxygen and glucose (blood sugar). Their nostrils flare and their breaths come in rapid gasps, with grunts or whines at the tail end. The muscles between their ribs retract with the effort; they appear even thinner than before. In short order their lips and fingertips become blue from lack of oxygen. Without help, their entire system is so disrupted in a few short hours that their arms and legs can swell with unmoving tissue fluid.

A baby so weak from the work of mere breathing hasn't the metabolic strength left to make surfactant. By taking over the vital functions of breathing and warming, and pumping essential calories into the blood, the machines of the NICU give such a baby a chance to rest. With rest comes the bodily strength to repair the deficit, and the cycle is often broken.

SHARON NAITO IS A SMALL WOMAN. SHE LOOKS EVEN smaller than she is because of the delicate bone structure in her face and hands. Her hair is black and rapidly going gray; her dark eyes peer through glasses. She speaks in a clipped, barely noticeable Japanese-American accent. Sharon Naito has been head nurse of the NICU for almost twenty years, a temporary promotion she accepted when her predecessor left in a hurry. Sharon found she liked the job.

"Nobody had intensive care, and babies just died," she tells me, perched on a rocking chair between two incubators. She doesn't rock, but sits as though in a straight-backed office chair. "It was basically well babies that were premature. We had sick babies, but they just didn't make it."

In those days, premature babies were routinely given oxygen in large amounts as well as prophylactic antibiotics. Fluids were given to those babies unable to drink by an almost obsolete method called clysis—the injection of fluid into the small layer of fat on the shoulder blade, to be slowly absorbed. As the evening nurse, Sharon cared for ten infants with the help of one nurse's aide.

At almost the same time as Sharon was enjoying her sudden promotion, the field of infant care went through an unexpected transformation. Two technical advances were most responsible for the shape of the field today. For the first time, respirators were made small enough and delicate enough for infants. Respirators to this day are essentially bellows—but so are the lungs. To keep from crushing the infant lungs as surely as a strong grip can squeeze a peach, the machines needed finesse in pressure, power, and speed. In the same heady period, new laboratory analyzers were developed that could examine certain elements in the blood using very small samples—the droplets that were all most premature babies could spare.

After an entire history of powerlessness, physicians had, at last, some tools. Instead of watching the infants struggle for breath, they could order respirator treatment—and with the lab machines they could begin learning what worked, what didn't, and what standards to demand from themselves and their charges. "Things really moved fast after that, all kinds of things," recalls Sharon. The unit was moved once, then twice, and again while the current ward was remodeled. Its size and staff more than doubled, and neonatal intensive care became a legitimate specialty for physicians and nurses alike. This particular hospital, long the community leader in care of the critically ill baby, hopes to find the funds to build not just a ward but an entire building devoted to labor, delivery, and nursery care.

The neonatal technologists gambled and sometimes lost. Some treatments that once seemed innocuous, even obvious, have delivered powerful and damaging blows. Lifesaving oxygen has been labeled the biggest villain, the traitor. It is extraordinarily volatile to a premature baby's flimsy cells: the pressure of the respirator-controlled breaths coupled with higher than normal concentrations of oxygen can make the cells of the lungs change until they become too large and airy to work. Oxygen is a sly element, and after years of being blamed for problems, it is suddenly getting off the hook—at least by some researchers. Retrolental fibroplasia—RLF—long considered the fault of oxygen, is now being laid to other treatments.

The newborn infant is a growth machine; the fetus more so. Every cell seems to clamor against the bit, begging to be released. If the small blood vessels to an area are constricted, it is a signal to the body to grow more. The body responds with a wild, immediate overgrowth of new vessels, producing weak, untrained capillaries that are quick to swell and burst with hemorrhage. For decades premature infants on high levels of oxygen have shown such changes; the results can be mild or devastatingly severe.

The overall condition is called retinopathy of prematurity; the term RLF is usually reserved for the more serious cases. Premature infants on oxygen are now routinely seen by ophthalmologists many times in the course of their hospital stay, and the minuscule growth and scarring of the capillaries in their eyes are recorded and followed. Mere vascularization, as it is called, is the milder form. Scarring, which contracts and pulls on the retina, is far more alarming: the retina of the eye is a finely balanced piece of work. Pulled out of place, it can leave the baby blind.

In the 1950s, RLF affected about 37 percent of the children at risk for it. Recent studies show the rate among RDS babies like Dale to run around 15 to 20 percent, although many individuals claim the rate is higher. One study of babies weighing between 700 and 799 grams shows a risk factor approaching 100 percent. Another, more recent study suggests that the bright lights in hospital nurseries increase the risk of permanent eye damage.

Many of these babies simply suffer from nearsightedness, and almost as many have a condition called anisometropia, in which the eyes see at different distances. Others have permanent squints or dim vision for no apparent reason, and a fraction have partial or complete retinal detachment. Such babies are treated with special glasses or eye patches, and many end up in surgery. New laser treatments bear promise for babies with weak or dragging retinas. Nothing cures RLF. Some babies simply go home blind. One out of five goes home with serious vision problems.

No one really wants to talk about RLF. High levels of oxygen were used for many years without thought of potential problems. It was lack of oxygen, after all, that killed the babies. A jury recently awarded $3.11 million to a ten-year-old girl who went blind during the course of her intensive care as a premature infant; ten years ago neonatologists were only beginning to understand how RLF worked. The blindness was blamed on too much oxygen, and the doctors were blamed for ordering it— despite the fact that much evidence now points to carbon dioxide and to metabolic disturbances no one is yet able to control. Eventually, RLF is likely to be laid at the feet of many elements in the care of premature infants, and some of the blame simply will be the fault of the infant's audacious age.

The vagaries of a premature system are so complex that the best management cannot keep every baby stable all the time. Environmental oxygen itself may be toxic to a baby's eyes, yet be insufficient to prevent brain damage in a baby not breathing well. If a baby's circulation is not working properly, it hardly matters how much oxygen is going into the lungs, because vital organs will still be deprived. Oxygen concentrations are now kept as low as possible for the shortest possible time—cost and benefit balanced on a scale.

IN THE BED NEXT TO DALE IS A FULL-TERM BABY BOY AS yet unnamed. During his birth, for reasons still unclear, he was without air for a few critical moments. He never breathed normally and then began having seizures. He is on a ventilator at very fast rates and very high pressures—high enough to risk rupturing a lung—and still his oxygen levels stay dangerously low. He is comatose from the barbiturates given to control the seizures and paralyzed from the drug given to prevent him from resisting the ventilator, which could cause bleeding in his brain. Monitors trail across his lap and chest and wind round his legs and arms. His TCO_2 monitor is covered with a tiny silver heart someone cut and pasted on.

This baby's brain wave is abnormal. At moments his brain seems to show no activity at all. Is it brain damage or the result of the drugs? No one is sure. He lies totally limp and sallow. The doctor pries open his eyelid and the pupil stares out blankly; the doctor lifts his foot and it hangs flaccid; then the doctor drops it with a tiny thud to the blanket.

Every new parent experiences a phenomenon commonly known as the "ideal baby syndrome." During pregnancy the mother and father both fantasize about the unborn child, imagining what its sex is, what its features will be like, how it will act and interact. Choosing a name for a person never before seen, weighing it against a feeling, the whole process serves a useful purpose, enabling the parents to move aside and make room. But then the real baby arrives, and regardless of his or her condition, no real baby can meet ideal expectations. The few weeks—and for some people, months—that follow the birth are spent melding the two, real and imagined, together.

How much harder this is when a baby is sick. Premature babies disrupt not only the expectations, but also the timing; literally no one is prepared for them. This anonymous baby was not early; chances are his parents had a name or two in mind, but they choose not to give it to him—it isn't his. His parents planned a home birth, and they stayed at home for a time even when the mother's labor failed to progress as hoped. From before this baby's birth he did not match hopes or desires. The white-sheeted rush of the ambulance and operating room—for he was eventually delivered in an emergency cesarean surgery —have only added weight to the difference.

Neonatologists, as well as the specially trained nurses

and obstetricians who work with them, all tend to disparage home births. They are trained to intervene; their workdays are spent with ill babies. As I rock in the chair between Dale and his neighbor, I can hear the terse comments and criticisms reserved especially for the parents of sick children who did not seek immediate professional guidance. The parents are presumed to be, at best, well-meaning fools. At worst they are cold criminals. Here is a perhaps unbridgeable gulf—a gulf of good intentions at cross purposes. The parents long for a baby to hold, and the baby can't be held. The doctors long for answers, a pellucid understanding. Doctors, I doubt it is so simple. I doubt the parents of this failed fledgling are cold.

The course of RDS usually peaks in twenty-four to twenty-eight hours and then begins to improve. Some babies may be acutely ill for several days, a few for weeks and even months as crises and complications pile on each other. On Dale's fifth day of earthly life, the attending physician gathers his four residents—all of them garbed in discreet khaki scrub coats—around Dale's bed to determine the next step of treatment.

"Is the respirator still helping him?" he quizzes the resident assigned to Dale's case. "Does he need it? Why don't we pull it?"

The resident hesitates, glances at the pile of neatly penciled graphs in his lap, and starts to speak.

"What I see here," says the attending physician, a small, sandy-haired man with thick glasses, without waiting for the resident's answer, "What I see here is a relaxed baby. Granted, he fought the tube a while, but he's not fighting now." He picks up one of Dale's feet and Dale sluggishly flexes his knee. "What I see is a calm baby, a baby who's breathing around the respirator as it is." He drops the foot and looks expectant.

The resident clears his throat: "We could start weaning him off, I guess." He looks enormously unsure.

The attending physician smiles impatiently. "Why not try him on CPAP?" [he says, referring to continuous positive airway pressure]. "His blood gases are fine. Let him do the breathing and give him CPAP at 30 percent instead of 25." He reaches over to the respirator controls. "That is, if I can figure out how this thing works."

A ventilator is a marvelous thing, capable of great variation on the theme of full and empty. The ventilator can breathe *for* a patient or *with* a patient, can deliver set volumes of air or set pressures, can allow a patient to take extra breaths in between or prevent him, and it can even control the way the lungs deflate. People commonly fight a ventilator, and they are sedated for their trouble. The fight can be disastrous. Trust the machine, the struggling patient is urged; everything is taken care of now.

Dale has been on "intermittent" ventilation, able to take a breath of his own, but required to take a certain number each minute. The machine has inflated and deflated his lungs for him at a certain rate, over and over, for days. On CPAP he will breathe completely alone, in full authority for almost the first time since his birth. But the positive pressure means that he won't be able to deflate his lungs completely. Take a breath and then let it out —now stop before you've finished and take another breath. Patients fight CPAP too, for it's not a normal way to breathe. Some say it hurts. As Sassall's patient explained, I suspect that ventilators and their various settings all sidle in where people live, insinuating themselves between the patient and the life-giving air, controlling what has long been a very private matter. It is an enormous loss.

Dale is being given CPAP so that his precious alveoli cannot collapse. If they did, they may not want to inflate again, and much of the surface area of his lungs would be out of commission. Time would be lost. The oxygen will be raised a bit, to 30 percent, and everyone will watch and wait to see what happens next, what Dale can do. The attending physician finishes twisting the knob, his students make notes, and the herd moves on.

Sue, Dale's nurse, leans on the cart beside the incubator and listens. She is a large and cheerful woman who has worked in the NICU for fourteen years, and right now she wears a grim smile. Babies are usually weaned off ventilators for at least several hours, sometimes days, before being made to breathe all alone. This transition is sudden and, to her, a little worrisome. She has spoken only a few words to any of the doctors, and then only in response to questions. Already the attending physician has hurried his brown herd to another bed, without a nod to Sue.

Within thirty minutes, Dale is wheezing. His breast-bone, soft and flexible, retracts deep into his chest with every breath, and the breaths come quickly and irregularly. Dale is struggling. Sue must go to lunch now or skip it completely; she asks the respiratory therapist to stay with Dale while she's gone. If Dale wasn't newly on CPAP, another new nurse could simply look him over now and again in that half hour, but Sue wants him to have one pair of attentive eyes.

Every two hours, on average, a technician arrives at Dale's bedside and draws a small sample of blood from his UA line. It is not uncommon for a baby to grow anemic from this slow drain. The sample is injected into a $20,000 machine—this unit has two of them—which analyzes its gaseous contents with certain chemicals and electrodes. Within two minutes the machine spits out a small piece of paper printed with the temperature, pH (degree of acidity or alkalinity), oxygen content, and carbon dioxide content of the blood. This is called a blood gas sample, and it is the statistical bible of the ventilator. Dale's TCO_2 electrode is a constant, but only general, indication of how well his circulation is pushing oxygen. The blood gas describes in no uncertain terms how well his lungs are absorbing the oxygen they are given.

W E GO TO LUNCH, SUE AND I AND A FEW OTHER NURSES, and we talk about Cabbage Patch dolls while we eat. When we come off the elevator into the quiet, empty hall, Sue is talkative and laughing. She washes her hands in the foyer and then stops short in front of Dale's crib. In the half hour she was gone, someone has pulled his breathing tube completely. He is off CPAP, off the ventilator that an hour before had completely controlled him. "Someone made a mistake," she whispers, but she doesn't mean it was an accident. The attending resident is a man of strong opinions and quick decisions. It was his decision.

Dale is wheezing, and now the muscles around his ribs are drawn in with each breath—"pulling intercostals," a classic sign of respiratory distress. The respiratory therapist covers Dale's face with a mask that blows medicated steam to open his throat and lungs, ease the tightness and swelling. No one speaks to the attending physician, who is far across the room and unconcerned. No one questioned the decision. The current opinion is that the ventilator should be used for the shortest possible time.

Dale's blood gases have dropped a little—less oxygen, more carbon dioxide. Dale is working hard for his air.

Sue, who says she likes her job better than anything else in nursing, says now, "I'll say something to him, I guess. Maybe. The doctors are in too much of a hurry." But she stays at Dale's crib.

Twice this afternoon Dale's heartbeat slows enough to cause an alarm, but he recovers on his own. More medication is added to his IV.

A NIGHT PASSES. THE NEXT MORNING THE ATMOSPHERE in the NICU is upbeat, jovial. It is the day of the cheesecake bake-off. Dale is still pulling intercostals, still sucking in his sternum with every breath, but his blood gases are better. He props one soft red foot up on the opposite thigh and meditates behind his bandaged eyes, joints flexible as a yogi's.

Four cheesecakes, each numbered for anonymity, are lined up on the shelf behind the desk. Dr. Art Eisele, the medical director of the unit—the boss—appears from nowhere trailing three medical students in green scrubs. They have been delivering babies. Nurses appear, residents gather, and Sharon Naito sits at the charting desk with a pile of papers.

Everyone lines up with paper plates and plastic silverware, and the contest begins. As we slice slivers of each cake onto our plates, the discussion centers on the merits of texture versus richness of taste. The presence of a chocolate cheesecake invites discussions of the importance of tradition. Crumbs spill on charts and people return for seconds; I sit next to Sharon, who pierces small bites of graham-cracker crust and chews thoughtfully. The votes accumulate in an empty bandage box.

Twice a baby in a nearby crib alarms. An intern looks over; a nurse peers at the intruding ventilators. The cakes are rapidly disappearing. When the dust settles, Sharon Naito wins the bake-off with a classic sour cream-topped recipe. She just smiles.

M ORE THAN OXYGEN AND ITS CONSTANT JUGGLING CAN complicate the babies' treatment. The first feedings must be gently handled lest the system be overloaded with fluid or the immature intestine shocked into irritation.

Babies can die from an unusual but uncontrollable condition called necrotizing enterocolitis, an inflammation of the bowel which kills entire segments of intestine and can throw the child into shock. Although not caused solely by feeding, enterocolitis is most certainly associated with it, and a baby in its grip cannot eat. In many cases the only treatment is to take the infant to surgery and cut out the dead portions of bowel, as much as is necessary.

Antibiotics backfire too. These drugs can cause deafness, stomach inflammations, permanent kidney damage; they can stain the hidden teeth. In a baby with a limited ability to fight bacteria, they can lead to "superinfection," infections caused by organisms resistant to many antibiotics. TCO_2 monitors can burn the skin. The electrode must be moved every few hours; Dale's slim chest sports bright red circles from past sites. The big concern, though, is always the brain—the brain and its tailing nervous system—and the damage that can follow a lack of oxygen in proper amounts or too much of this and too little of that.

A ROUND THE CORNER FROM THE CHARTING DESK, IN full view as you enter the foyer, is a bulletin board filled with pictures of unit "graduates" labeled with name, birth date, and birth weight. These are snapshots of happy little children playing on the beach or whooping it up at a birthday party. Some are four or five years old now, those who weighed only a few pounds at birth; these Polaroid snapshots serve as a constant silent reminder of what is possible.

Not every graduate, however, gets his or her picture on the board. Each nurse and doctor I speak with privately remembers certain children. The same ones. I hear the same stories over and again, from people eager to unburden themselves. The stories are about children who survived, but who are profoundly retarded, crippled with cerebral palsy, blind or deaf, or all these things at once. Everyone remembers a happy couple whose marriage fell to shreds, a successful lawyer who became an alcoholic, the mother who still comes to visit three years later carrying her two children who cannot yet walk or talk—the mother who says that if she'd known, she would never have allowed it to happen. Some NICU graduates are in institutions and will likely stay there all their miracle lives.

"It hasn't been too long—five or six years—since we used to sort of have an unwritten rule that any baby under so many grams wasn't to be intubated," says Sharon Naito. "First it was 1000 grams. Now we intubate 600 grams." Intubation is the opening of the airway, of a door—ventilator treatment. The borderline, she remembers, just gradually shifted downward, a few grams at a time, as technology and the skills of doctors and nurses improved. Sharon thinks that any one baby's chances are the result of a number of characteristics and that simply looking at age or weight is not enough. "It all depends on how they look when they're born, even; it's not just weight and gestation sometimes—it's just how strong they are when they're born. Because some of them are just born like they aren't going to make it. They look like jellyfish."

The majority of surviving RDS babies are normal, although most suffer from delayed emotional bonding to their parents and the developmental delays common to premature babies. The sicker the baby, the longer the delays. Many complications, such as abnormally weak muscle tone, tend to improve in time. But every group of survivors in every study in the literature has abnormal children in it, some with pulmonary problems, vision deficits, hearing loss, emotional disturbances, and neurological problems. Cerebral palsy and retardation are not uncommon at all.

Lozano reports that 30 to 40 percent of the very premature infants who survive have IQs under 90, below normal. He reports "severe" neurological problems of different kinds in 18 to 54 percent of survivors. Another study, though, of the very small infant under 800 grams reported a "remarkably hopeful" outcome with very few severe problems of any kind. But this study and others like it must be read carefully; 80 percent of the babies in this range died and were not included in the "hopeful" outcome. The authors of the study point this out dutifully, without irony. The babies who were really bad— who had hemorrhages in their brains or whose brain waves were distressingly abnormal or weak—were taken off treatment. Their ventilators were unplugged, and they died. These are the babies who would have skewed these "remarkably hopeful" statistics to a less positive reading. In other words, if your baby is not so sick as to have treatment suspended, he or she has, perhaps, a better than fifty-fifty chance of beating retardation or cerebral palsy or its kin. The alternative is no treatment at all. Who decides?

D R. ART EISELE IS A LARGE, FLORID MAN IN LATE MIDDLE age. He slouches in chairs, and a little smile plays just at the corners of the large mouth in his big wrinkled face. Eisele keeps his counsel until he is ready to speak, listening with what almost appears to be amusement to those around him. When he begins to talk he doesn't finish, even if he must interrupt, until he has said his piece on a subject. Now he is talking about the future and the borderline that has steadily dropped gram by gram.

He points out, as have many, that it is the lung that matters most, not the age. Gestational age is different from a simple chronicle of weeks and months. It is a question of fitness, not time. "There'll be an occasional baby at twenty-four weeks, just because of biologic variation, that may have a chance at survival," says Eisele. But in the critical period, survival means not only unusual vigor but "hundreds of thousands of dollars of intensive care and everything else."

Recently a group of investigators reported on their use of a new machine called ectracorporeal membrane oxygenator—ECMO—in severely ill, very young newborns. ECMO is a variation of the heart-lung machine used in major heart surgeries. It is a crude artificial placenta that bypasses the intense resuscitation of the lung for the natural, fetal, version—arteries and veins. Blood flows out, is filled with oxygen, and flows back in, mechanical, mother to child. The infant still breathes, if he or she can, but the lungs needn't be efficient. The infant needn't struggle; it can lie in the warmed bed with its little monitor and dream baby dreams, dream about floating again in the dark waves. All that's missing is the whoosh of the mother's heartbeat.

The physician's are positive. In one study, forty-five babies who were unable to survive on ventilators were put on ECMO; twenty-five survived and twenty of them appear normal. In another study, twenty-two patients were put on ECMO, and 68 percent survived. And in the latest group, of nine babies on ECMO, six survived and five, for now, appear normal. Take your chances—four out of five, five out of six who make it, and the occasional one who doesn't. How to weigh the neatly wrapped parcels of pain? Here is hope, for those who seek it, that the boundary of age and gestation can keep shifting ever downward, pushed at the opposite end by in vitro fertil- ization. The womb made obsolete. ECMO makes me un- comfortable, the way a Bosch painting or crooked room makes me uncomfortable. It doesn't fit; something is out of place, missing, broken.

"It would be a fantastic, fantastic expenditure of time, effort, and money for what I think would be a continuing massive experiment, and with a large number of people coming out of it not being normal, not being right, having brain damage, this or that problem," says Eisele about ECMO. "It would be this constant problem of knowing when to stop. It's opening Pandora's box in ways that I think we would look back on and say, 'God, this hasn't been worth it. We've spent billions of dollars and what have we got? It doesn't make sense.' Even though you can technically do it for a while doesn't mean you nec- essarily *should* do it.

"The natural thing would be to let the baby die and let the family go on and have a chance at having more normal children. It is so unfair to them as human beings and to this baby as a human being to do all this with an outcome that is experimental, so chancy, so unlikely to be satisfactory—that we're playing with them as humans."

He is concerned about the power of physicians and nurses. He frequently brings up "people's expectations" of him and medicine itself.

With all these complications, these man-made trials of error, with outcomes, as Eisele says, so chancy, people might begin to wonder. Should we be toying so with ba- bies? Should we perhaps take a deep breath and consider a moment? But the outcry has been of quite the opposite kind—for greater interventions, for the machines to be used when even the physicians and parents are unwilling. Lucky Baby Doe.

President Reagan's Department of Health and Human Services recently unveiled what may be the last set of regulations aimed at controlling the treatment of sick newborns. The Baby Doe controversy has continued for three years, since the time of a single case in Bloomington, Indiana, in 1982. That baby died, lending its anonymous name to the whole problem.

The Baby Doe regulations require that physicians provide all available treatment to all infants with only three exceptions: babies who are in comas with no hope of emerging, babies who must inevitably die despite all treatment, and treatments so "extreme" and so likely to be in vain that they would be inhumane. This last is surely the trick, for all along that has been the explanation of the physicians and parents who would withhold treatment to certain babies—but withhold it not because of the treatment, but because of the baby. The courts are full of contradictions, but they have many times upheld the truism that only life, and not the quality of life, can be considered in treatment decisions. "This is premised on the theory that life is the ultimate value, and something to be preserved regardless of prognosis, regardless of cost, and regardless of social considerations," writes John Paris, who clearly doesn't like the idea.

Some hospitals have met the rule by assembling committees, hopefully composed of thoughtful outsiders, physicians, and nurses who can be called upon to decide the best treatment for a particular child when the parents and physician disagree—or in those difficult situations in which members of the community "blow the whistle" on physicians and parents who have quietly agreed to stop treatment. The Baby Doe regulations and their resulting myriad analyses are, to one committee, "a flawed and ill-defined set of rules under which physicians are to perform their medical duties without due regard for their ethical and legal obligations to their seriously ill newborn patients and their parents." No one is happy.

The new regulations are no more likely to solve the

problem than the old ones, no more able to define words like "extreme" and "inhumane." The words, in fact, are necessarily fluid. The parents of Little Boy Blue, in the bed beside Dale in a coma and with an abnormal brain wave, think he is receiving extreme treatment. They had hoped for none at all. His physicians, in turn, think the parents acted inhumanely by delaying medical care. This difference is not as much as it first appears to be, with words like "extreme" and "inhumane." It is a difference of purpose, of desire. The parents see the treatment as the flexible factor—that which has changed and can be controlled. The doctors see the treatment as a standard, a model, unwavering, growing ever more refined. The baby is the equation's mysterious, unpredictable factor X. But the tables twist and turn. The first time the Baby Doe regulations were invoked against this hospital, by a small but vocal group who had heard a baby was not being given life-saving treatment, the baby they wanted to save had been born with its brain completely outside its skull, hanging from its head in a silky sac.

No one wants to reach across and flip the switch. Baby Doe rules require that someone must, eventually, because they require the switch to be turned on in the first place. "I panicked once in the air, when I thought the patient was going to die. I knew the patient was going to *ultimately* die, but I didn't want the patient to die with *me* in the air." These are the words of a nurse who works in a flying ambulance, gathering up the children too sick to be treated in rural areas and returning them to the city and the uncommon machines it holds. She sees babies and children die many times a month, and still slides away from it, alarmed. This power, this unique fragile demand, should be given to those who have never seen it before.

Sharon Naito will schedule her uncertain or disturbed nurses away from such babies. She thinks the nurses bear the heaviest burden; though they are unable to make the decision, they must listen to the parents' grief and carry out physician orders that may be most disagreeable. Eisele has a method of his own for sorting out the different sides. If, against all odds and against his recommendations, the parents want treatment to continue, he'll continue. But if parents want to stop treament in spite of medical hope for recovery, he'll override their wishes. He tries to err on the side of hope. Many babies, the majority of those who die in the NICU, die from not being given more treatment when they worsen rather than having treatment withdrawn. "We draw lines all the time," says Eisele, "and obviously some of the lines are arbitrary."

As I began these stories I suggested a morality—a possibility—with which to face the labyrinths of our own making. One facet of such a philosophy must face the problem of power and helplessness, for that is an essential problem of illness. Here in NICU it is a most acute and disconcerting problem, but one no one names. Power? Here, where so much effort, time and money are given in the altruistic urge to save life? But the very smallness of the patients, which makes people feel generous, also makes the discrepancy of the power unavoidable—actually physical. This is the root of much of the indecisiveness and, ironically, of the aggressive confidence. When it comes to the fate of people so obviously lacking in control, how else to act but with a hearty certitude? If nothing else, we might bluff our way out.

The lights in the NICU are so strong, the shadows so stark, it is sometimes hard to see the shades of gray. An understanding of power and helplessness in this context must include the knowledge that *both* parties, patient and caregiver, have strength and weakness. We see that the patient is helpless. He is in danger of being overwhelmed; his attention is solely on his deficits. He is dependent— he has surrendered. But caregivers, no matter how long the strides, are helpless, too. Even if we can change the course of the disease for now, we can't change anything for good. We can't control the individual, eccentric course of anything at all—we can't make the patient behave. All this mad fumbling with the controls is also a thumb in the dike. Sometimes we know that, and sometimes we forget. Everybody dies.

The pitiful little patient has power, too, even when he weighs a measly pound or two. He has the power to embrace and accept what grips him, whether it is life or death. He can initiate his journey to health, accept or reject the assistance offered. We know the power of the caregiver. What has been missed is how intricately and intimately patient and caregiver, power and helplessness, are entwined: it is our very prowess and machismo that makes the caregiver feel so out of control; it is the patient's valiant defeat that gives him the power of passive resistance. And, in turn, it is passivity that mystifies us all. In it lies the mystery and the fear of what comes next. Round and round we go.

Before it is born the baby has power, too. She bobs slightly, tilting her head; in photographs the light transilluminates her skull and its delicate tracery of circulation. We gaze dumbfounded at these pictures, of the human too brittle and glassy to survive. The mother of this baby moves to catch the hiccuping motion of her belly while she looks at these pictures; at another time, the same woman would long to be rid of the possibility that grows inside her. She would beg for deliverance.

The smallest babies in NICU, the monkey-faced, skinny ones that can't be held—they are abortable by law. Such late abortions are far more uncommon than the vocal opponents of abortion would have the public believe, but they happen. Whether they are an unfortunate necessity or a brutal tragedy depends on one's viewpoint—on one's condition, so to speak, in relation to the artless pictures. Babies are brought to birth stillborn and defeated or welcomed with the blaring of mechanical trumpets, depending on expedience and sorrow. How the skilled specialists and trained nurses will react to any single eggshell-frail infant is, in the end, a matter of context. Some of these nurses and physicians or their close companions have had abortions, and they come to work prepared to save the lives of babies barely bigger. In a way, for many, abortion is irrelevant to this work, however odd that seems. Babies—and all people—are endowed with meaning according to how we see them, how they will change the way we see ourselves.

ART EISELE IS MORE THAN A NEONATOLOGIST; HE ALSO sits on the board of the local Planned Parenthood. He has, in fact, written a speech about abortion from his peculiar point of view. He says it is truly not for him to decide. Put the child in his care, lay it on the table, and he will fight for its life; anything else is out of his control. He strays from the subject of abortion, which in an important way is irrelevant to his work. He would rather discuss the need for prenatal care for low-income women, the young, and poorly educated women who have turned for solace to abortion so often in the past.

AS USUAL, THE ATTENDING PHYSICIAN WILL BE VINDI-cated. His gamble has paid off, saving him a bit of time. Dale is on room air, breathing lightly, easily, just three days after the ventilator was stopped. His drugs are done. Today a tube will be inserted down his mouth to his stomach for his first meal. Sue says nothing.

His neighbor, the unnamed boy with an odd brain wave, is faring poorly. His circulation is so erratic that much of the air being forced into his lungs is leaking into his skin and muscle tissue. He is blown up like a toad, puffy and soft. His blood gas oxygen is far below normal, indicating continuing damage not only to his brain but also to all his oxygen-dependent organs. He shows no signs of con-sciousness, even with the drug doses lowered, no ability to breathe without the ventilator. His parents have been approached once about the possibility of turning the ma-chine off. The boy cannot recover; he won't suddenly blink and start to cry. Each person who watches can't let his held breath go. After all this, his parents have changed their minds. Keep him going, they say, suffering. What have we done, they wonder.

This is high-stakes poker, this NICU. Just to buy into the pot is a major investment for most families. The bed alone is $630 every day. The ventilator is extra; the drugs, diapers, syringes, ultraviolet lights for bilirubin, the ox-ygen monitor, and the heart monitor—all extra. It costs money to start an IV, to draw a drop of blood to check the number of red blood cells, to catch the stream of urine to check for sugar. Blood gas samples, which are taken ten, twelve, sometimes fourteen times a day, cost $42 *each* time. A week can easily cost $10,000. Most families cannot even consider paying such costs, and the bills go to welfare or insurance or are left unpaid. NICU is a big loser for the hospital, looked at in black and white, but such so-phisticated treatment brings in more than its share of federal grants and loans, foundation money, and research projects. Technology attracts experts and the best staff, and even in the tightest, most competitive of economies the ability to provide a type of care no one else can provide brings business.

"This country's medical system is so screwed up!" Eisele snorts. "We have all these marvelous things that people don't have a chance to get because they don't have the money; there isn't the organization for it. We have to remember that all this wonderful stuff here is bankrupting families right and left. It's great that we get all teary-eyed about how much good we're doing, but we're also devastating people's lives as the price for this."

Eisele believes in national health insurance. Between 30 and 35 percent of the patients have no source of money whatsoever. That's a lot. The part of the population that has no insurance, no health insurance, is a part of the population that tends to have premature babies."

Research developments continue, quietly. For years steroids have been used before an inevitable premature birth, given to the mother in the belief that the drugs could speed up the baby's lung development—but the results are discouraging. Eventually an artificial surfactant, now in the experimental stages, will be available to spray or blow into a premature baby's lungs and, hopefully, prevent the development of RDS in the first place. Each success and every failure is a wealth of knowledge —what worked, what didn't. Each baby is a clue to a staggeringly huge puzzle.

A group of physicians in St. Louis has attempted to reduce the number of babies with brain hemorrhages by paralyzing them. They theorize that the devastating bleeding—which, when severe, causes retardation and cerebral palsy—was partly related to the struggle of the infants' to breathe, when in truth the ventilator was breathing for them. The lack of synchrony, the disharmonious pressures of baby and machine, disrupted brain blood flow. So the doctors paralyzed the babies, just as Dale's neighbor is paralyzed, and then the babies just lie there, resigned. Of fourteen babies given this treatment, nine are normal several months later—two-thirds, compared to 40 percent in the group receiving "standard treatment." These are the odds; ante up.

All things considered, though, neonatal mortality is dropping steadily and has been for many years. A problem common to all medicine is that all these follow-up studies, discouraging or hopeful, are based on last year's technology at best, but, more often than not, on the technology of five years ago. If someone suddenly sees trouble, he can't yell "Whoa!" until thousands of babies have passed under the bridge he's waving from. Today's methods, today's approaches, are wholly untried, their long-range effects unknown.

Eisele says that the most important advance would be "making available what we have in ways that are not going to injure people as much as help them—and injure them in the broad socioeconomic sense. It doesn't require any fancy technological breakthrough." I think he is the lone voice yelling "Whoa."

A BOUT A MONTH AGO I WAS WORKING FOR THE EVENING on a floor called the Mother-Baby Unit, where new mothers come soon after delivery. Their infants usually follow, in wheeling, plastic-sided beds with little cupboards underneath for diapers and T-shirts. I was caring for three mothers and two babies; the third baby was upstairs, in the medium-risk nursery. After supper I peered in at this boy's mother, just to check, and saw her shaking in bed, crying, clawing at the sheets with her eyes squeezed closed.

"I want my baaaby!" she cried, rolling back and forth,

tugging at the IV tube in her arm. "Get me out of here!" She wept a long while, certain her roommate, whose baby was also upstairs, had hidden an infant somewhere in the room to spite her. "I heard a baby cry, I know it!" she insisted, to me, to the head nurse, to other mothers walking by.

Later that same night I telephoned for the pediatrician on call because I was worried about one of the babies in my care. She seemed like an FLK. I had a feeling with little to support it. But for hours there were no pediatricians available—everyone was gowned and gloved, sterile, excitedly preparing for the imminent delivery of a twenty-three-week-old premature infant. Hours after I called, a resident appeared. She was brusque, impatient; she flipped her neat brown ponytail out of her way when she talked. And watching her I realized something.

The nurses coo to the babies. Male and female nurses alike, when they reach in the crib to lift the newborns, begin to sing. They purse their lips and squint their eyes and turn every word into an extended vowel, whether changing a diaper, cleaning a face, or pricking a heel with a sharp blade for blood. The nurses coo, and the doctors don't.

This resident confidently flipped the baby over, ran her hands surely over her head and skin, pinching here and measuring there, peering in eyes and at gums. The baby began to cry; the doctor was quiet. More than quiet: she was silent. It was then that I realized that I'd never seen the doctors in NICU or the nursery sing to the babies.

She took my little FLK upstairs, and I perched on the mother's bed to try to explain. Tests, observation, don't worry. I know you've just delivered and you're shocked by the power and strength of new life, but don't worry. Baby is in good hands now.

TEN DAYS AFTER BIRTH DALE IS BUNDLED UP FOR THE ride across town, to a neighborhood hospital close to home, adjusting to feedings in less rigorous circumstances. Sue puts on her coat; she'll go along for the ride. The bed next to Dale is empty again; this morning the ventilator was turned off and, with his parents' final, sad blessing, the unnamed baby died.

TRIPTYCH

TONIGHT IT'S MY TURN TO WORK, IN THE INTERMEDIATE-care nursery of another hospital. This is a halfway house, a stopping place on the way home for premature and sick babies. Some infants graduate from the NICU to come to intermediate; others begin here and work their way home. The room is at one end of a long hall filled with pediatric beds, tucked in a corner where the hall turns, with windows looking out. People automatically peer in as they pass.

It's a warm, clear April Saturday evening, and I'm responsible for two babies. To enter the ward, I must stop at the linen cart outside the door and cover my clothes in a hospital gown. So garbed, I meet my wards. Mine is an easy job, simple vigilance, as I watch two healthy premature babies grow a day older.

Li is a Chinese boy, weighing in at 3½ pounds; his head is covered with slick black hair. He sleeps, skin sallow

59

against the faded crib sheet. Brian, his next-door neighbor, is bigger at 4½ pounds, obviously plumper—a pale, blond baby. I can see at a glance that he is cranky; he holds his face in a tense prune. Both rest in high cribs, bundled in flannels, and both wear three-lead monitors.

They are good breathers for such little creatures so early out of the sea. As the night wears on, I find that the monitors are peevish things: sometimes they sound the bugle call for an apparent reason, but usually the alarms are due to the simple wail of discomfort—an angst alarm.

Two of the remaining three babies are also premature. Their nurse arranges her time like mine—much of it is spent in a rocking chair.

Li and Brian are notoriously picky eaters, quick to vomit. I coax fractions of ounces into tender stomachs, whispering encouragement into crooked ears. We do our best, with bottles and nipples specially designed for tiny mouths and weak cheek muscles. A few ounces of formula get down every few hours, with naps between. Li wants only to sleep, and I wake him rudely, again and again, unclip his wires and bounce him softly into my lap. "Soup's on," I smile, and he settles uncomfortably into the hollow of my arm, for all the world like a workingman awakened too early on Saturday morning.

In the far corner of the room, with a nurse all her own, is one last baby. She is full-term, well-developed. When I stand over her crib for a peek, I am struck; she is a startlingly beautiful child. Her name is Janelle, and she has a myelomeningocele.

WE HAVE GREAT FORCES AT OUR FINGERTIPS; GREAT forces work all around us in the dark. Take a chance; nothing's certain anymore.

Myelomeningocele is a fancy abbreviated term for a

ghastly defect, one of a set of conditions called spina bifida. The error begins in the very first weeks of life, when the fetus is floating in a syrupy fluid, barely formed and silent. At this tender age, ontogeny is recapitulating phylogeny; like a pollywog, the unborn curls in a crescent, its arms mere flippers, its frog legs drawn casually close. The spinal cord forms first in the center of this germinating seed and grows both ways, up to the top-heavy, translucent head and down to where our tail was millennia ago. Most of the time the cord grows straight and true, and then the vertebrae form, encasing the cord in a strong and flexible tube of bone.

At times, however, some part of the bone fails to form. I am one of the thousands of people with spina bifida occulta—that is, the back of one of my lower vertebrae is missing. But my spinal cord lies in its hollow undeviating, as it should. Looking at me, nothing seems wrong—and really, nothing is. Except for that odd gap on my x-rays and a few misaligned vertebrae above, I am fine. And lucky.

Without its cage, the cord can curl up outside the skin in a delicate cyst of spinal fluid and milky membranes. Myelomeningocele is a severe type of spina bifida. The cord and its nerve fingers tentacle out and twist round in a blemish perched on the back, a great shiny, bloody balloon of a blemish as big as your palm and an inch high. It swells out like swamp gas, like a lava bubble threatening to burst.

Every 800 births a woman is delivered of a child like this, unbidden and shocking, its spinal cord open to the harassing, dirty world. What happens then depends on several circumstances. Often, much of the damage is already done: paralysis, retardation, misplaced hips. The height of paralysis depends on the position of the sac of spinal cord; it may affect the legs, the trunks, or even the arms. The bowel and bladder are often paralyzed too, flaccid, so wastes dribble constantly. The spine may be twisted sideways or up in a hump, the hips may be out of their sockets, and the feet may be clubbed, atonal muscles pulled by healthy ones above into odd shapes, taking the bones with them. Nine out of ten myelomeningocele babies are born with hydrocephalus, in which the cerebrospinal fluid accumulates in the brain and the head swells, sometimes monstrously, pressing on the fragile brain and crushing the cells. The eyes bulge out in amazement at the unexpected pressure.

Certain diseases become metaphors, such as cancer or leprosy. They wreak a kind of devastation on the body that seems more than simple-minded cell growth, more than misfortune. They seem to be symbolic of the larger condition, of humanity's changing states. Myelomeningocele, in a subtle way, has also been made into a metaphor. It is an example often used for better or worse in arguments about the fate of ill and ill-made babies. More than one Baby Doe has suffered from myelomeningocele. The injury can cause such extensive damage and guarantee such permanent crippling that even the most conservative textbooks discuss—albeit glancingly—the possibility of withholding care. Rather elaborate systems have been developed to determine the probability of a quality life for a baby with a myelomeningocele, and many neonatal units have practiced a kind of unwritten, random protocol for treating some babies aggressively and others with simple supportive nursing care. One of the tricks of myelomeningocele is that, although devastating, it may not be immediately fatal. With many of the worst birth defects, even the most zealous pediatrician hasn't a hope in hell of saving a child's life. Myelomeningocele babies, though, can surprise you.

Whether it is for the benefit of any casual observer who may happen across them or for the less-conscious needs of the writers themselves, the words used to discuss this problem are illuminating. To delay surgery is to open the door for death, but this is said very formally, very carefully. I have a book that states, "There are those who recommend that surgical repair is best delayed for further assessment of neurologic function, intellectual potential, and extent of complications." I open another book and find: "The decision of whether or not to treat must be made before neurosurgery is undertaken, since closure of the defect assures at least temporary survival." In these sentences, held at arm's length ("there are those . . ."), is such confusion. It is a veiled anguish that we can't discuss. Most of us see a baby like Janelle and see our own weaknesses and failings so clearly; we see our selfishness. We see her and ask only that the cup be taken away from us.

B RIAN IS UNHAPPY. LIKE SO MANY HE IS ANXIOUS AND easily stressed; this is a tough, bright world. The slightest disturbance and he cries for comfort, for peace; he has *weltschmerz*. I pace with this fretful one who sends the monitor running for cover. His head rolls on my shoulder, but when I lay him flat, he howls again. We pace more, and I have time to watch.

Janelle's nurse busies herself over the dressing, an intricate swab of medicine and gauze pads. It is significant that this baby is already named, not like the puffy-skinned boy in NICU. Many parents, staggering from the blow, withdraw from their errant child and cannot call it by the name that a few days earlier had rolled so lovingly off the tongue. Janelle's wound opened in the lumbar area, high above the soft concave curve of her back. She is paralyzed from at least her chest down. She has yet to move an arm or hand. Her head has begun its inexorable swelling, and tomorrow a shunt will be placed in her skull to drain fluid off her brain and deposit it harmlessly in her abdomen. She may be quite retarded, and with every hour the damage increases, brain cells popping one by one.

Spina bifida, in all its forms, tends to run in families. With one child like Janelle, parents must count on the possibility of more—a four to eight times greater chance. The luck of probability doesn't hold in genetic gambling. But medical science holds out a tempting choice—the defects of spina bifida can be detected by amniocentesis. A needle plunged into the amniotic fluid surrounding the developing fetus can be used to remove a few cells. Such cells are examined microscopically for shape and placement of the master genes—which shell is the penny under in this game? The test is done around fifteen weeks of gestation, almost four months into a pregnancy, and results come more than a month later.

Writing about prenatal diagnosis, one researcher blithely states: "With these techniques, many congenital malformation syndromes can now be diagnosed at mid-trimester and prevented." Through his entire discussion, this doctor never uses another word to describe the abortion he is advocating. He is concerned with preventing birth defects, not with aborting a fetus in the fifth month of pregnancy.

As soon as Janelle's dazed parents were able, they gave permission for surgery—to slit her back and slip the cord in place. Without surgery she would quickly have gotten meningitis, which would very likely have killed her. Without immediate surgery—within a day or so of birth—she would not have been "assured at least temporary survival." The first door is opened and closed; this one locks behind you. Writing about the dilemma of treating these babies, an ethicist suggested: "The basis of selection for treatment in cases of myelomeningocele ought to be the presence of a commitment by the parents to care for and nurture their afflicted child."

A young woman, still a teenager, enters the nursery with a flourish, tying her gown behind her as she crosses the room to Brian's crib. She introduces herself to me when I stand to hover over his crib where he lies sleeping at last. She is his mother, Linda, thin and all nerves. She scoops him out and bounces him around the room, talking. It is an hour before he is due to eat, and he shows no signs of hunger. Despite my suggestion against it, Linda opens a new bottle and settles down to feed him. She has little success with the tired baby whose stomach is still nearly full, and she rocks rapidly in the chair while fussing with the nipple, talking to no one in particular without pause.

At the height of the evening we have a new admission to our small room, necessitating the movement of cribs, the rearrangement of chairs and monitors, the making of room. Sarah comes in a high, hot Isolette; she is not yet 3 pounds, but she's a day old, wrinkled, red, and simian. Even the veteran nursery nurses crowd round her to coo and moo. She sleeps on, eyes clamped tight against the bright light, naked but for a diaper smaller than a table napkin.

F OR THE CHRISTMAS OF 1984 THE CABBAGE PATCH DOLL manufacturers, ever eager to catch new levels of tolerance, marketed (with success) a new model, the Cabbage Patch Preemie, hairless and pink and bulbous-faced. I wonder what is next. Big-skulled hydrocephalus dolls? Cleft palate babies? Perhaps a twisted-limbed spina bifida. They could call it Baby Doe.

I am sitting in the chair with Li, wiggling the nipple in his mouth to remind him of our mutual goal. A young couple appears at the window. Their faces are blank, composed. The man—tall, handsome, and mustached—wears a yellow baseball cap emblazoned with the name of a trucking company. He helps the short, plump woman into a hospital gown outside the door. She drapes it over her clothes and smooths it down. He follows suit; then he reaches for the baseball cap at the last moment, pulling it off in a crumbled fist like a farmer entering church. He stands shyly by the door, a young man in jeans and button-down shirt dressed incongruously in a hospital gown. She moves at once to Janelle's crib, to her daughter.

Because of the surgery on her back, Janelle must lie on her belly and be moved on a board that enforces her prone position. Of course, she cannot be breast-fed; the angle would be impossible. She is changed prone, fed prone. To lift her, her mother must lift the whole board. She cannot curl her up in her arms or cradle her. The nurse helps her balance the board on her lap, Janelle spread before her like a feast. Her husband moves to her side and scrapes a chair up, embarrassed and polite.

Brian's mother talks on in the background, and I look at Janelle's mother. She is beautiful, pale, full of face, tired. Her dark hair hangs round her face, which emanates a sweetness grown brighter by the ordeal of a long labor and the violence following. She keeps her expression calm, tranquil, running one hand lightly over Janelle's hair, softly, softly, without pausing, speaking to her in psychic whispers. Occasionally she confers with her husband, and they nod their heads together, seeking comfort one from the other. They are an island.

The essential myth of Baby Doe is that parents who choose to forego aggressive treatment for their defective baby are heartless and unloving. Surely such a myth is comforting, blending as it does all shades of gray into simple black and white. The baby, clearly, can't be wrong. No baby can be wrong. Therefore, the parents are; they are cowards. They choose the easy way out.

All choice is hard. To choose not to do is hard. Janelle's parents—have they any idea, any idea at all, about what they are getting into? Have any of us, merrily whistling in the dark down these echoing corridors?

Brian's mother announces her exhaustion and rises to leave. I offer to take her son, whose feeding time and discomfort have now arrived. Linda stretches and yawns, asking if it would be all right if she went home to sleep now and didn't return till morning. Yes, I assure her. She gathers her bag and leaves.

I feed Brian, also with little success, and change his diaper. Time for tests. I take his wet Pamper across the hall and squeeze it until a few drops of urine fall into a test tube. With a simple chemical, I check it for sugar to ensure the stability of his metabolism. Li has a diaper changed too, a bottle, and is patted to sleep, relieved to be left alone.

Brian cries and screams and trembles. Anyone will collapse in a few days with an irritable baby, and I wonder about Linda's endurance. A half hour after he falls into slumber, she returns with relatives in tow and wakes him so they can see. He fusses and won't smile despite her exhortations. The room is suddenly crowded and noisy. I am as annoyed as if she had grabbed hold of my own sleeping baby. Linda is determined to hold court and speaks loudly to the room. "He's never been so cranky before," she tells us. "I had a friend," she says to all. "They said her baby was going to be retarded. Can you imagine that?" And she shakes her head. My heart sinks. Janelle's mother smiles politely, nods her head. She strokes and strokes.

As the evening wears on, I see the ripples in her smooth expression. Her face works with great subtlety; she begins to learn her new life. She is sorting out dreams, discarding ideals, reshaping the corners and crannies for Janelle's distortion. It is not just the physical world that must be adjusted to fit Janelle; that is easy enough in comparison. Both mother and father must be made to fit her too.

The chaos settles. Linda, nervous and haggard, tightly wound, leads her kin out, and with effort I get Brian back to sleep. When all is quiet, I go to find the head nurse and tell her my concerns about Linda. She lacks confidence, knows nothing of baby care. She is just a girl. When Brian is strong enough to go home, she will expect him to perform in certain ways: it is a textbook family for child abuse. It is all I can do. When I return to the room, Janelle's parents have left. I never learn their names.

We gather our charts and note accounts of the evening almost done—how much drunk, how much spit back. When the writing is over, we circle our chairs protectively round the cribs and talk. I discover, in passing and trying to disguise my interest, more about Janelle's parents. They are children too, as I suspected—she is seventeen years old, he a year older.

Janelle could have been worse, after all. I have spent more than a few hours in the dim library stacks of the medical school, turning pages of color photographs, stark nightmare after stark nightmare. Here is a baby with rachischisis, her entire spinal cord and brain exposed to air; the child is irreparably split from forehead to tailbone as though with a cleaver, a fleshy fissure of a baby. Here is a cyclops, an infant boy with a tiny head puckered and fused in the center, and with only a blank, fatty bulge for a face. And here are the twins, melded together like wax on a hot stove, a leg here, two arms there, with no head between them. I turn the pages on my own preoccupation with these sorrows.

THE MYTHS OF GREECE AND ROME SPRANG OUT OF OUR fascination with form—centaurs, chimera, Pan. Perhaps these ill-shaped babies, born early, usually dead, manifest our own unspoken, unrealized demons, the impulses we keep locked tightly away. In the Darwinian world, we turn away from them for a simple and eminently practical reason—to get on with the business of the species. These distorted misconstructions, lacking faces, limbs, breath, are not human—but neither are they less. Evolution makes its jerky, mysterious gains in just such ways, and the mistakes left behind have much to say about our obsession with form. Every culture has its snakes, born full-grown from a woman's breast, but we've cataloged them, latinized them, and filed them away.

What a riddle. Look, we have saved Janelle's life, she is a miracle! It is motion as swift as the embroiderer's needle, patch and darn. Her mother, pretty angel, casts aside a fantasy and opens her arms to accept what is given. Is this the difference, then, between prevention and elimination, between Janelle and a monster? Do we grant humanity? Is it ours to take away?

What a wonder, how we are given the children we receive—the injuries and the sorrows we receive. Here is another riddle, science. It is like the lottery—you stand in line for a ticket and the person in front of you gets the winning one. If only you'd found a parking place sooner. So many eggs, so many sperm, so many tiny bacteria and parasites and planes that crash. Decisions that last a lifetime, made in the small moments of between-dreams.

SISTER MEAN

ONE OF THE MOST PECULIAR COMPLICATIONS OF OUR health care system is the quantification of suffering into money spent and money due. It has been long remarked on. The equations are sorely berated and carefully examined, we shake our heads and keep on filling out the forms. We shake in our boots, too, staring down death, and all the while wonder how much the whole thing is going to cost.

The economist Lester Thurow pointed out in an article in a medical journal that when it comes to expensive medical treatment, Americans have inconsistent ethical systems, being both capitalists and egalitarians. "As egalitarians, we feel we have to provide the treatment to everyone or deny it to everyone; as capitalists, we cannot deny it to those who can afford it," he writes. "But since resources are limited, we cannot afford to give it to everyone." Ah, dilemma, the niggling discomfort of entitlement programs, government's well-meant protection of those in need. We are torn between that grand satisfaction of giving to those in need (a bit abstractly, at arm's length) and the more immediate security of expecting each to pay his or her own way.

Medical entitlement programs, though—and Medicare is the greatgranddaddy of them all—have two other characteristics that our inconsistent ethics fail to resolve. First, entitlement is not unlike the respirator that breathes for the comatose old man: it's so much easier to start it than to stop it, so much easier to do something—anything—than not to do. And once it is begun, in all good intention, an entitlement program cannot be stopped without consequences similar to those when turning off the respirator: someone will die and it won't be the person flipping the switch. Treatment freely granted becomes a right fully expected—a matter not of preventing, but of terminating.

There are also the forgotten effects of the treatment itself, the suffering that follows *getting* the treatment. The treatments picked up by special programs are often the more exotic and unusual, the technically sophisticated, and are aimed at specific conditions—precisely what makes them so expensive that they require entitlement (and it is the entitlement, more than anything, that takes them from the exotic to the ordinary in our minds). In contrast, a school lunch program for poor children or free prenatal care for pregnant women is too dull for words. But a school lunch program is arguably free of serious side effects and unexpected grief. Technical medicine is not.

In this world of egalitarianism and capitalism, where falls compassion? No one has asked, away from the cameras, away from the courtrooms and legislative hearings, how it feels to be permanently tied to a breathing tube, nor what it is worth, in terms other than money. We all pay for it, wrong or right. State legislatures vote to fund a particular small child's liver transplant or experimental chemotherapy program, and a hundred more send in their requests. Enormous intensive care bills are shunted to the welfare system, or simply written off by a hospital, which then raises room rates to other patients. What are we paying for in the name of equal access? Into this murky entanglement falls the end-stage renal disease program, for many years the example, the precedent, of what good intention can bring.

"For I have moved closer to death, lived with death," sang Theodore Roethke. He might have written those words while he watched his blood flow in tubes beside him. Dialysis is a game of machines giving way to better machines, a game of blood and waiting. The renal dialysis patient is always waiting, half well, half-sick, birth child of modern medicine and noble desire.

S HE AWOKE WITH A SORE THROAT ON A SPRING MORNING in her third year of college. Molly was twenty years old, contented and athletic. She went to the infirmary and a throat culture was taken; she was told, a few days later, that she had strep throat. A minor, not uncommon inconvenience to a college junior. Molly had rarely been sick, had never had surgery, but she took the prescribed penicillin willingly.

She didn't get well; she got worse. Molly began running fevers and feeling weak, lethargic. Her muscles ached; she lost her appetite, lost weight. After two months Molly was still taking penicillin, her strep throat stubbornly refused to improve, and she was sick enough to be put in the hospital. A few weeks later she lay in intensive care. Only then did a doctor recognize the trouble—Molly was allergic to penicillin. But the damage had been done. Her kidneys were ruined, severely injured by her reaction to the drug.

One day in midsummer, a nurse brought a dialysis machine to her bedside. "I didn't know what was going on; nobody knew, really. They just had to dialyze me, my kidneys weren't working. I'd had so many IVs and machines beeping and buzzing all the time that—I looked over at the machine, and it was *huge*, the dialysis machine—I said, 'Oh, that's just another machine, I can handle that.' " Without explanation, the nurse fastened a needle in Molly's arm to the tubing on the machine. "It was all red, all this tubing was all red, and I said, 'What's that stuff?' 'That's your blood, Molly.' 'All that is *my* blood?' I passed out."

Molly is one of over 71,000 Americans on kidney dialysis. More than half are under sixty-five years old, and the population increases every year. Fifteen percent of these people will not survive the first year. Molly has a lot of company, more company than anyone imagined a decade ago. Though hardly a "major" health problem in terms of the numbers affected, kidney failure, dialysis, and kidney transplants cost the Medicare program almost $2 billion a year, with no end in sight. The Great Society goal of equal health care for all has gone awry.

Beneath the cheerful nurses' voices, the mechanical announcements of the intercom, and the beat of the rain outside is a pulsing hum, an alternating current of sound, oscillating, artificial. It sings almost below consciousness, seductive; you pat time to it internally. This hum is never absent. Late at night, when the last patient has left, I know the machines are turned off, but I cannot imagine the silence that is left.

In this large room with closed doors, labeled KDU (for Kidney Dialysis Unit), is a flattened horseshoe, an arrangement of leather armchairs and hospital beds, each place separated from the next by a machine. Long, looped yards of tubing dangle from the machines and run through spinning pumps and electric eyes, following a guided trail. The tubing is filled with dark red blood. Attached to the ends of it, feeding it, are people.

The horseshoe faces a bank of televisions hung from the ceiling and wired to earphones. The silent color pictures flicker in the fluorescent light and reflect milkily on the steel of the machines; the shiny white light in the room makes the late afternoon rain outside seem darker, bleaker.

Tonight the beds and chairs are filled with the members of the Monday-Wednesday-Friday evening shift, Molly's group, one of six groups of patients whose lives center around this room. Molly is propped up in the hospital bed in the center, facing the nurses' desk where I make my notes. Joe, midtwenties, is silently watching the news with his lips parted and earphones clamped round his ears. In the hospital bed next to him lies an old man, sleeping; the man's wife sits beside him and holds his hand. Another patient, Nora, very short and elderly, greets everyone as she enters, even me, a stranger. There are so many strangers here. She settles into an armchair; she is so short her feet dangle off the floor. As I move to a chair beside her she is struggling with the top of a red-plaid coffee thermos, a new *Time* magazine in her lap. She smiles at me and calls out to the nurse nearby. "I sent away for this hair-restoring remedy. What do you think?" Her mousy brown hair is thin, frizzy. "You're a sucker," laughs the nurse, and just then Nora pops the top off and the coffee spills down her front. I get up to find a towel.

Above an empty chair, splashed on the ceiling, is a scatter of old blood. The week previous a tube had come unhooked and sprayed its rhythmic arterial pumping across the tiles, the ceiling, the patient, and several nurses. Such minor crises are not uncommon, and neither are the major ones. Tonight the sleeping man—terminally ill with cancer—is in the process of "crashing," his blood pressure dropping dangerously low as the blood volume shifts with the dialysis. A nurse hovers near him, taking his blood pressure every few minutes and adjusting the machine.

This is a singular and select population, these dialysis patients. They come to this room three times a week, for three or four or five hours at a time, and sit down to be stuck with needles and drained. Each would die without the treatment, and a little over a decade ago they would have had no choice. Dialysis is a technology that has guaranteed uncertainty and confusion; it has given life, temporary life, to a class that is condemned to death. Each is a "marginal man," not well, not quite dying. Now this class is condemned to wait, for one technology has to breed another. The "renal community," as it calls itself, has had machines, and then better machines, but the chance for life without a machine seems a long way off.

W E DON'T THINK MUCH ABOUT OUR KIDNEYS. WE RISE from our seats and plod into a bathroom several times a day, giving the process of urination little attention. It's a nuisance, this endless business of washing out wastes. Kidneys are unassuming characters, but they keep us alive in an orchestrated dance of water, salt, hormones, and poison. The kidneys produce substances essential to the making of strong bones, healthy and adequate blood cells, and stable blood pressure, and by their balancing act, the heart beats on time. When our kidneys are healthy, we can abuse them—overloading our systems with fluids and then again with salts and minerals, depriving ourselves of water and nutrition or gorging on protein. Through the loops of Henle and the proximal tubules, in Bowman's capsules and the labyrinthine glomeruli, through 1 million nephrons in every kidney, our circulation quietly trickles, all day and all night long.

But the kidneys can turn suddenly rotten and ruined, swell or shrink, grow fat with tumors or scarred and cramped. Kidneys are subject to cancer, cysts, infections, and the crystallization of thin, sharp stones, and they suffer dearly from the effects of diabetes, high blood pressure, and just plain age. A surprising and disagreeably long list of drugs—aspirin, many antibiotics, drugs for seizures and tuberculosis, anesthetics, and many more—are nephrotoxic, that is, "kidney poison." Those noble kidneys, though, can help keep us alive even when 99 percent of their function is lost, so a failed kidney isn't usually removed. It just hangs there, dripping a bit of urine or hormone now and then, marginal like the person.

People in the first glimmers of kidney failure may notice only that they have begun getting up in the night to urinate. Their urine becomes pale, straw-colored. Their feet swell. They lose their appetites and then begin to vomit from a nausea that never ceases. Their skin itches madly all over. Edema, that spongy cushion of water under the skin, rises up their legs, chest, and arms, and gets behind their eyes, until their vision dims. They taste a bitter metal in their mouth; their breath is fetid, fishy, almost ammonia. Their feet burn; it feels as if there are bugs crawling in their legs. No position is comfortable. Men become impotent, women sterile. As time passes— and how much time depends on many things—a uremic frost covers their bodies until their skin turns orange-green or gray. Their hair is brittle and falls out in handfuls, and they bruise at the slightest touch. They get nosebleeds. This is uremia, urea in the blood. Urea is a nitrogen compound, a poison, but it is not the apparent source of the symptoms. There is no one clear-cut villain in uremia; all we know is that it kills.

By now, such people are nearly dead. Their blood pressure is too high, their bones are too weak and porous, their blood is thin and anemic, and their minds are confused. The calcium that's abandoned the person's bones has deposited itself about the body—in the arteries and eyes and heart. Death comes from the heart stopping, too much potassium.

Some types of kidney failure are temporary. Acute failure can come on in a matter of hours and is a life-threatening emergency. Sometimes it can be corrected. For chronic renal failure—known as CRF—medicine offers no cure, no replacement for the delicate cells of the nephrons, nothing but the hum of the machines and, for a few, dreams of a transplant—the better machine.

"Dialysis" means diffusion, the movement of particles from an area of high concentration to an area of low concentration, across a membrane. Kidney dialysis can be accomplished by filtering the blood across an artificial membrane—hemodialysis—or using the person's own peritoneal membrane, a drape of tissue in the abdomen. Hospital-based hemodialysis is the method that serves 80 percent of the population.

Hemodialysis machines now stand about 4 feet tall and almost an arm span in width. Ten years ago they were almost as big as an economy car and about as loud. The tubing is draped intricately on the exterior along a carefully charted course beginning with the patient's artery. Blood flows into a filter, a long, light tube about 15 inches long and the diameter of a flashlight. This filter is the dialyzer itself—the artificial kidney. It is filled with thousands of tiny hollow threads made, most often, of a plastic similar to cellophane. A dialysate solution surrounds the threads, and as the blood drips through the threads, waste molecules and excess water pass through the membranous cuprophan. The composition of the dialysate and the speed of the pumping can be changed to increase or slow down the process, temper side effects such as nausea and cramping, and maintain blood pressure. Patients call it "pulling." The waste dialysate, spiked with uric salt, ammonia, proteins, sodium, and much more, is pumped into the body of the machine and then discreetly drained into the hospital sewage. One drop of blood passes through the dialyzer in less than a minute; the blood goes round and round, in and out of the person's body and the artificial kidney, for hours and hours until it's clean.

On average, a filter costs $26, and is thrown away after one use. So are the yards of tubing, the unused mixed diasol, the leftover bottles of salt solution, and the needles and pads. Between patients, the nurses clean each machine, taking down and setting up equipment, cleansing its inner workings through the rarely silent pump.

How, one may ask, does all this blood get in and out, day after day? "I've had about eighteen surgeries on my arm," says Molly matter-of-factly, holding up her bruised right arm. One day, she recalls, she was in the unit over twelve hours because they couldn't get a good vein. "They had to stick me thirty, thirty-five times." Access—to arteries and veins—is the ogre of hemodialysis. "I think it's the greatest source of stress for most of the patients," says a nurse. "They don't sleep at night worrying about how they'll get stuck the next day."

Molly's surgeries involved the insertion of a shunt, a flexible tube between an artery and a vein in her forearm, because no one's blood vessels can stand up under the repeated needling. The gentle curve of the shunt bulges against her thin, pale skin, too delicate to hang a purse over. It is into this fortified vessel that the needles are stuck, a buttress against bruising and clotting. A new fistula (a word for an unnatural connection) swells and aches and cannot be used for months. In the meantime, other vessels in the leg, abdomen, and chest can be used. The needles are bigger than you expect, short and stout, without the fine, half-invisible point that lends a bit of reassurance to the routine injection. They are tiny knives; they cut through the skin and the abused veins. The nurses inject a little Novocain before they wield the blade, like dentists homing in on a tooth.

As an experiment, a few surgeons are working on something called the "button," a shunt that comes above the skin so that only the plastic need be sliced. It is a problem beset with technical difficulties, but it can be done. I asked a vascular surgeon why more aren't done. "Too expensive," he said. "They cost $3000 each. Medicare's not going to pay for it, and none of the patients are willing to put up the money." Nor is this physician, who sets the price, willing to lower his fees. He feels he is not adequately reimbursed for his time as it is.

Dialysis is not safe. Patients crash. Infection at the access site is a constant risk, as is uncontrolled bleeding afterward. CRF patients tend to have anemia, poor blood clotting, and a subnormal ability to fight infection, yet as a group, they are exposed to far more risks. Hepatitis is a constant fear, and units can have epidemics of it in both patients and nurses because it is spread by blood; the bugs can find a corner of the pump to hide in and never be found. The tap water in many cities is high enough in aluminum and certain minerals that chronic dialysis patients have been found to have toxic accumulations in their bodies from the dialysate mixes. As a consequence, most units have special, expensive water filters built into the plumbing system.

Almost half of all dialysis patients are hospitalized at least once a year for treatment of complications of either the disease or the dialysis, and 10 percent are in the hospital four to ten times a year. With the best of treatment, only half of a given group of dialysis patients will survive five years. These extra costs aren't considered in the costs of dialysis, which in 1983 was about $26,000 per year for each patient.

M OLLY RESTS IN A HOSPITAL BED NOW FOR HER THRICE-weekly flushings, relaxed and confident, if not happy. She knows the slang and talks casually about access and "getting on" the machine. Her thin, freckled face and casual hairstyle belong on a woman five years younger than her twenty-six years; her dry, wrinkled skin and gaunt, bony figure belong on a woman three decades older. Molly hasn't always been a "well-adjusted" patient.

After her first few dialyses, the doctors decided to wait, putting her through the process only when it was absolutely necessary, hoping that with time her kidneys would regain enough function to keep her off the machine. She became too weak to walk, lost more weight, and felt herself slipping into a lethargic depression. "I wanted to die—because that would have been easy," she recalls. "Everybody was doing everything for me; I couldn't feed myself because my arms were just tied down with tubes. I was on oxygen. I just didn't care anymore." Molly had always been a little afraid of needles and blood. Now she found herself inured to constant, painful pricks and her own blood flowing before her eyes. Her jaded reaction frightened her more than anything else. It's not "normal" to be used to such things. Was she no longer normal?

Eventually the physicians relented and told her she would be on dialysis the rest of her life, or until she received a successful transplant. For the next six years she was too sick to consider surgery—often nauseated, weak, fighting infections and the side effects of the dozens of drugs she received. A person in kidney failure has an extremely difficult time metabolizing drugs and suffers complications and toxic reactions with alarming frequency. Yet Molly managed to finish college and find a job. She says now that Norman Cousins' book *Anatomy of an Illness* "turned her mind around," and she became determined to beat the bad blows she'd been dealt. "When I got back to school, I had lost all my hair from the medication, and it was just growing back and was kind of fuzzy. I didn't care. Mom wanted me to get a wig, scarves, stuff. I said, 'Mom, if people can't accept me for who I am, then they're not even worth it. That's the way it is.'" Returning to an "ordinary" life was not easy. Molly wondered if she was sexually normal: "Hormones are in the blood, and dialysis washes the blood, right? So I wondered if it washed out my female hormones." She gave speeches on dialysis for her communications class. When she lost her first job because of extended sick leave, she simply found another.

Optimistic writers claim that a life as independent as Molly's—dialysis schedules aside—is possible for many CRF patients. Nora, the elderly woman with the thermos, is too old to be considered for a transplant. Yet she went on a cruise to Alaska this past summer on a ship with a dialysis machine on board and a nurse trained in the process. Molly has achieved her successes through a measure of assertiveness that many people resent in a patient. She is suing the doctors who failed to diagnose her penicillin allergy, admits she is "picky" about who sets up her machine, and has told the head nurse to keep certain nurses away from her. The surgeon who does most of the shunts in this unit openly dislikes her. He says the disease is "her own fault," and that she is trying to avoid responsibility for herself. During her sessions she speaks up for the quieter patients, relaying their requests and calling for assistance for her neighbors. She is granted admiration almost grudgingly by the nurses, and a bit of resentment as well. But no outward accomplishment, no job or degree of outspokenness, makes life on dialysis normal.

CRF patients must immediately and forever change their ideas about food. Every bite of anything, every sip of fluid, is potentially harmful, even lethal. Every patient is different, depending on age and size and condition, the illness that led to the kidney failure, and the degree of function left. Each person requires more or less of salt, water, protein, calories, vitamins, and minerals. The blood levels bounce around like dented Ping-Pong balls, erratically and unpredictably. A patient's weight can change by 20 pounds in the day between dialysis runs.

For all but a very few, the first thing to go is salt. No more potato chips, pretzels, popcorn, and soda crackers. Say goodbye to lunch meat, lox, bacon, sausages, hot dogs, pickles, mustard, relish, and Chinese food. Never a pizza, taco, antipasto, olive, or bite of sauerkraut. No molasses, nuts, canned soups and vegetables, TV dinners, or peanut butter. No cheese, not even cottage cheese. No seasoning with soy sauce, no dried fruit. In extreme cases, even foods with baking soda and baking powder are taboo— no bread, biscuits, or bagels.

Many must avoid phosphorus, so they give up milk. (Just as well, it's too high in salt.) But they also have to avoid chocolate and whole grains. Potassium is commonly withheld; a potassium overload can cause a heart attack —so that's the end for yellow fruits and vegetables (yams, bananas, raisins, avocados, tomatoes, broccoli, and potatoes). Some people must restrict their protein, taking in half the normal amount; 2 ounces of steak and a couple of eggs will do it for the day. Yet this same person may need 2400 calories a day, almost twice the normal requirement. If fluids are restricted—and they usually are—melting foods such as jello and ice cream are withheld. Not easy for someone who may have to swallow thirty or more pills a day. What does this person, this teetotaling Spartan, eat? Candy. White sugar. Oil, lard, and butter. Low-protein amino acid supplements. The CRF patient, because of the disease, tends to suffer from hyperlipidemia, the "fatty blood" condition we're told can lead to heart attacks—and to prevent which we avoid candy, sugar, oil, and lard. A rock and a hard place. In an effort to make even more out of the diet, researchers are attempting to perfect "keto analogues"—the ultimate food source, honed to its nutritional parts, synthetic. Unfortunately, by all accounts, keto analogues taste bad. Compliance is a problem.

Partly out of simple appetite, partly out of a need for control, dialysis patients frequently break their diets, sometimes with little treats, sometimes with long binges. A binge can make renal failure patients very sick; it can even kill them. To avoid this responsibility, such patients will blame someone else—often the nurses, harping on their techniques or their mistakes. They may blame the machines or claim that the lab tests were inaccurate, knowing all the while what they had for lunch. Nurses can be exceedingly sarcastic when they talk about their noncompliant patients, stuck between a protective urge to hover and their own need to blame and chastise. No one here is going to get well, period. No one is even going to feel all that good, no matter how skilled the nurses or how well-adjusted the machines. The diet is the turning point of control, of push and pull, of who's in charge.

A nurse tells me privately, with surprising vehemence

in her voice, "I'm sick and tired of people saying it hurts when they dialyze. It only hurts if they cheat."

A S MANY AS TWO-THIRDS OF THE PATIENTS IN A DIALYSIS unit suffer a psychiatric or psychological illness. About half are unemployed, either because of weakness, depression, or a dependence on the public assistance that would be lost if they got a job. Dialysis patients, many believe, come to their illnesses with an unusual burden of mental illness in the first place. Without a doubt, dialysis serves a group of people who are affected by the poverty cycle: poor nutrition and health, lack of health care, lack of education and employment, and poor prenatal care set a person up for the debilitating illnesses that often lead to renal failure, and once on dialysis and into the Medicare system, their continuing poor health and public assistance keep the cycle running.

The incompatability of free-market capitalism and egalitarian social programs is abundantly clear when the benefits go, as they often do, to people for whom capitalism has failed to keep its promises. For people who have never had money, never had success, never had a ride on that intoxicating merry-go-round of one victory and bit of progress building on another, entitlement grants them the rewards (a few specific rewards, at least) all at once. "All of a sudden, by an act of Congress, they not only have a physician, they have a nurse, they have a dietician, they have a social worker assigned to their case," notes a nurse who trains dialysis patients at home. Why jump off *that* ride to try to make it on your own? It never worked before.

Dialysis requires patients to be independent and dependent at the same time. The dialysis center is often the only social outlet, an outlet that will be lost—and not replaced—if a transplant is successful and health is restored. Family and friends expect the patient to get well and go back to work once treatments begin, but even with treatments the person rarely feels well. After months, perhaps years, of being relegated to the status of a sick person, half removed, it is not easy to return to the demands of routine life. There is no border between home and hospital, health and illness, surrender and victory. A machine, strangers, an alien tube bulging against the skin of your arm—constant reminders. And the diet, always the diet.

Compliance is a big word in the dialysis literature. The writing takes on an almost whining tone at times, an air of complaint, when discussing the difficulties of getting a patient to stick to the rules. Obedience is demanded, but dependence is discouraged. One must act well, but be sick; work and care for oneself as though healthy, but eat and schedule one's time as though ill. The independent patients, the ones who turn around and make demands themselves, are a constant irritant. They are the least easy, even when they are the most healthy. They are "difficult." They fail to surrender; they want more than the physical rewards of entitlement. They want to be whole again. They want respect.

This is not to say that all who make demands are simply making a statement of independence and spirit: some are simply off kilter, out of touch. One morning, as I sit at the desk with several nurses, a former patient calls from another state. I can only hear one side of the conversation, but it's obvious from the nurse's rubber-faced expressions, her eyes rolling and her mouth pursing, her mimicking to the other staff, that the caller is saying something interesting. When she hangs up and says the name, everyone nods and smiles in sudden understanding. "I'm just glad she doesn't live *here* anymore," grins the nurse who spoke with her. "She just called to inform us that she'd never had renal failure in the first place, and the whole thing was a big government hoax!"

All this feinting, all this alternating thrall and freedom, makes every relationship layered, every interaction pregnant. The intricacies of power are vivid here. J. Perkins Ellis, writing about his many years on dialysis, pointed out how odd and heavy were the nicknames given by the nurses to the dialysis equipment. The pumps were called such things as Killer Rabbit, Silver-Tongued Devil, and Cottonmouth. The dialyzers themselves were Shaft, Octopus, the Phantom, and Sister Mean.

Molly told me about an incident that happened to her in the first few months of her dialysis. She was young; it was a trivial moment. But in remembering it, remembering the way one particular physician treated her, she still grows angry, animated. Her eyes open wide, there's new life in her voice.

Molly had been told by someone that because the machine took care of her blood imbalance, she could eat whatever she wanted right beforehand. She sent her mother out to buy a longed-for enchilada, and just as she prepared to dig in, the physician walked in the room and took it from her hand. He said that she couldn't risk the chance of infection from food prepared outside the hospital. But before he left, he stood by Molly's bed and ate the enchilada while she watched.

AFTER SEVERAL DAYS AND EVENINGS OF VISITING THE KDU, talking to patients and nurses, poking through supplies, and peering at the machines, I was aware of a curious ambivalence between the nurses and their patients. Why do nurses, so many with backgrounds in emergency nursing and intensive care, come to dialysis, with its routine schedules, chronic population, and repetitive chores? So I ask, and they talk for hours.

The first reason I hear, from nurse after nurse, is the machines. The mound of metabolic detail and chemistry that must be learned, the complexity of the machines, is unusual for nursing. On-the-job training is a struggle; most nurses say they need six months in the unit to begin to feel comfortable. But therein lies the reward: the satisfaction of competence, of an esoteric skill, of constant troubleshooting and responsibility. Many of the staff want a break from the stress of intensive care nursing and think KDU will be, as one put it, "a piece of cake." When they realize it's not, they either quit within a few weeks or stay for years.

Another reason I hear, mingled with complaints about paperwork, is that dialysis nurses are spared much of the "drudgery" of nursing—the linen changes, bedpan emptying, and baths, those demeaning and unpleasant chores robots might someday spare us all. The nurses, working in a closed, often forgotten, part of the hospital, have an unusual amount of independence. They must get along with and take orders from only a few physicians, rarely seeing the parade of residents and interns that passes on other units. They are paid better than many of their peers—$12 an hour in some areas, as much as $18 or more in certain cities.

Still I see this ambivalence. Each patient is recognized, greeted by name, treated as an individual. Their histories and personal problems are known to all the staff. In a hospital, it is unusual for a nurse to get to know patients as well as these nurses know theirs. But in private, whether in the coffee room or in a low voice at the nurses' desk, hidden by the constant hum of the machines, the nurses are bare in their irritation. Not a single patient is without faults also known to all. They defend them and chastise them in the same breath. At a time when nurses have successfully won labor contracts guaranteeing them no rotation between shifts, the KDU nurses gladly switch from morning to afternoon to evening, and even odd days weekdays and weekends, so that no one nurse will be caring for the same people every day.

There are alternatives to hospital-based hemodialysis. Some people can be trained to perform hemodialysis at home, but such an elaborate setup requires "free labor" —a relative or friend who can be trained to assist day in and day out, week in and week out, for life. Because over a fourth of dialysis patients are single, such labor is hard to come by. The labor also must be willing and able to insert needles every time.

In recent years, peritoneal dialysis, the original method, has regained favor. Not everyone can use it—diabetics, for example, often have a dramatic loss of vision on peritoneal dialysis. But home dialysis of either kind is cheaper. Yet in 1983 there were still four patients coming to hospital centers for every one on home treatment.

Peritoneal dialysis involves the permanent insertion of a catheter in the abdominal space, and the diasol is injected into the hidden spaces between organs to slosh around the intestine, behind the bladder and stomach, while the membrane itself acts as a filter, pulling out body wastes and excess solution. After thirty minutes or so, the solution is drained away and the process repeated. Traditionally, the technique is used for several hours every few days, but a new method has become popular in recent years, called CAPD—for continuous ambulatory peritoneal dialysis. A person on CAPD is always dialyzing, always either injecting (a twenty-minute procedure), draining (twenty minutes more), or going about business with a bellyful of fluid—a few quarts for the average adult. You make love with it sloshing inside you, billowing up into a cushion. The whole process, in and around and out, is repeated four or five times a day. The advantages are its simple, low-tech feel, the independence from a hospital or machine, and its cost—a third less than the center. But many people feel nauseated constantly, and there is a consistent low rate of peritonitis that kills a few and hospitalizes others. Molly wouldn't consider CAPD or any form of home dialysis. "Twenty-four hours a day you're dealing with it." She points to the room of machines. "This is my little space, my little time to deal with this, directly. And I can go home and leave it here, most of the time."

The "suitcase" kidney makes a splash in the papers now and then. It is all the bulk and humming glory of the dialysis machine in the size and shape of a briefcase. Only a few are available, and like every technical advance that will free the patient from the hospital, it requires a motivated, bright, and relatively healthy person to use it. Any experimental advance will likely be reserved for the younger, healthier patients, the ones who are most likely to benefit, to be good statistics, to provide the encouraging data that bring in more research money.

Dialysis has created a population of thousands who can't be healed, who are too old, too sick, too depressed or worn or lonely to care for themselves. Dialysis entitlement—the government's ESRD Program—has created an expectation that this population can have no bounds, that this population will be kept alive, in whatever condition, as long as possible. Who can say no now? Who can turn off the machine while the blood runs, warm and fluid, in the tubes? Other chronic, incurable populations wait their turn. Millions of Americans with Alzheimer's disease have no financial resources for their care, no insurance, no veteran's benefits, no coverage from Medicare. The clamor is beginning to be heard: Who will pay for us?

National health insurance, with one flat rate and everyone guaranteed treatment, has long been heralded as the solution. But perhaps it's too late for that now. Medical research has given us so many new treatments, so many options, and the most expensive are the ones that don't cure, but keep sick people going, going, hoping for the cure to come. National health insurance won't work unless, as Lester Thurow suggests, medical professionals themselves are willing to say no to the idea of every treatment for every patient. It is the miracles of medicine in all its specialties that ensure that the old and sick fraction of dialysis patients will grow the fastest. It is precisely this fraction that will never use a suitcase kidney, that will never have a chance at a transplant, the almost-routine kidney transplant that doesn't work nearly as well as the public tends to think.

THE FIRST "SUCCESSFUL" HUMAN KIDNEY TRANSPLANT took place in 1954, after decades of experiments. Thirty years later 6112 transplants were performed in the United States—accounting for less than 10 percent of all dialysis patients. (In the 1940s, in an effort to stop the rejection process that was so obvious but so poorly understood, transplants had been followed with whole-body x-rays, the patient laid out and illuminated.)

Each person carries on his or her sixth chromosome— our miniature selves, our replicants—a chemical called the major histocompatability complex (MHC), which determines, more than temperament, more than persuasion, our likeness to another. It is the MHC which recognizes self and spies other, the MHC which lovingly accepts the growth of our own cells and vehemently repels the growth of foreign ones. Out of check, short-circuited, we mistake self for other and suffer "autoimmune" diseases such as lupus. Out of control, we suffer allergies.

A particular weapon, the antigen, is designed for each enemy and lingers in the body long after victory, waiting for its singular chore. The same is true of others' bodies that is true of a cold virus or grass pollen: a transplanted kidney is just a piece of meat where it doesn't belong as far as the sixth chromosome is concerned.

The solution to the problem of rejection lies in two parallel paths: to find organs so close in form that they "fool" a recipient's body or to find a way to prevent the antigen reaction to the organ in the first place. Parts of the MHC can be detected in blood cultures, as well as subtypes of these parts. Our genotypes can be laid out like fingerprints, fed into a computer, examined, calculated, and spit out in a permanent record. Needing a new body part, we look down the list for a likely donor.

As the children of two parents tend to share a subtly familial look, so do they share a tendency toward similar tissue types. About one of every four of a person's siblings will be a near match, two of four less so, and one no better than a stranger. An identical twin is almost, cell for cell, you. Trade kidneys and bone marrow like coats and blouses, fool the neighbors, fool the body.

A bad match is not just likely to fail; it can kill. The body defenses grow in urgency until often the only way to protect the patient is to remove the donated kidney and nurse the person back to a kind of health. But even a good tissue match is no guarantee. Immunity is a fickle and unpredictable thing, and it can be upset and confused by such procedures as blood transfusions, which are common to the CRF patient. Although the statistics are poorly kept and incomplete, a generally accepted figure is that ten years after the operation, only slightly more than half of all transplant recipients are still alive.

Having end-stage renal disease is not in itself enough to qualify a person for a transplant. There are not nearly enough kidneys to go around. Every transplant team has criteria of its own, differing from place to place and more or less flexible. The generally accepted criteria required to be placed on a list for transplant include age under sixty-five years (fifty-five in some places), no major cardiac problems or related diseases such as vascular disease (and in some centers, diabetes), freedom from infection, freedom from any sign of cancer for at least a year—sometimes five years—and either no history of drug or alcohol abuse or clear proof of rehabilitation. Every center looks at psychosocial criteria as well.

No part of medicine is free of the concept of selection criteria, however subtly it may be presented. On the one hand, looking at the statistical risks and benefits is a safeguard, a way of protecting patients from unnecessary, expensive, and perhaps painful or dangerous tests and treatments. If a person is at risk for a complication from a test—say, an angiogram to determine the status of the coronary arteries—then the supposed benefits should outweigh the possibility of problems. But because any cost-benefit analysis is based on statistical data and every body of statistics includes the minority number, there will always be people who are denied a treatment even though it would benefit them. No one knows, resources are scarce (especially other people's organs), and research support is based on positive findings. So a few—who knows how many—become sacrificial lambs. Unless and until we are willing to provide every treatment to every person, damn the numbers, a few will die from lack of a treatment someone thought might hurt them.

The real problem, the problem faced in the choice, is defining an "objective" criterion. Can age really be called objective when a person in his sixties may actually be in better health than a diabetic twenty-five-year-old?

Can we look at race? Blacks make up twice as big a fraction (24 percent) of the dialysis population than of the population as a whole; one possible reason is the higher occurrence of high blood pressure in blacks. When we turn away a person with a chronic illness or alcoholism, claiming that the risks are too great, we are actually stating that a limited resource—kidneys—should go to the healthiest people, and there we tread a fine line. Alcoholism and chronic illnesses are also often at the heart of the kidney failure in the first place. In the end we look at psychological criteria: personality, character, cooperation.

Until the costs of dialysis and transplants were picked up by the government in 1972, equipment and money were so scarce that participants were selected by committee. The losers died. The choices were based on both physical and psychological characteristics; the latter included "ability to cope with stress and to tolerate frustration . . . and the presence of a responsible family member willing to help in the care."

Such Hobson's choices shunned the poor who had no relations, those who had sought therapy, and more subtly, the nonconformers, people who demonstrated a penchant for questioning authority or demanding control. Compliance behavior meant a lot. No one is turned away from dialysis anymore, not for age or psychosis or disease, because the federal government pays, but they remain an obstacle for transplants. Why give a precious and fragile organ to a person unlikely to follow the regimen to keep it healthy? Why throw it away while a young, intelligent, adjusted person waits on dialysis, getting sicker each year?

The trouble is that the criteria were never very good at predicting success. Harriet Mercer is a registered nurse and transplant coordinator with the Northern California Organ Bank. She's been fooled more than once. The least likely candidates will blossom with a transplant. Others, long compliant and cooperative with dialysis, are unable to follow the rules that a successful transplant demands. Still, Mercer and her colleagues have a list of criteria—

even though they will talk to anyone interested—against which to compare candidates.

These criteria don't always measure the psychological problems created by a chronic, lethal disease or years tied to a dialysis machine. Most long-term dialysis patients have a less than ideal mental outlook. One study correlated length of survival with "marked indifference to fellow dialysis patients." Several studies show that the more a person denies the seriousness of his or her illness, the longer he or she lives. The blind eye to others as well as to self seems to serve these chosen patients well.

But say you're a lucky one, relatively young, healthy but for your kidneys, and you've led a clean life—nothing for the record anyway. Then the obvious best match is a healthy brother or sister. Waiting hooking up every other day, knowing your sibling is walking around with a good tissue type and two—count 'em, two—good kidneys can put a strain on a relationship. "A lot of the time there may be pressure on the person from everyone else in the family," says Mercer, especially if the sibling doesn't really want to donate. "We don't like to lie," she adds, but if a family member can't go through with it, "we may indicate that there's a problem in their physical exam to get them off the hook." In one study of people who donated kidneys to relatives, 15 percent felt "a little pressure. They believed that if they had not agreed to donate, their families would have regarded them as cold and uncaring." Donation is not risk-free. By going under the knife and giving one away, however altruistic or confused the motive, you lose your leeway. Your leftover kidney will enlarge, get more efficient, and you'll never notice the difference. But you are at higher risk now for someday ruining that one remaining organ and submitting yourself to the machine.

Molly is a lucky one; her sister Lily is a near-perfect match. Lily's reaction began as wholeheartedly enthusiastic, but as Molly's health dipped and rolled, she had time to reconsider. She wanted to have a baby. "She was really scared about that," says Molly. "About having only one kidney and having a baby—what would it do, what were the risks, the percentages, all that stuff. It kind of hurt." Molly began to think about cadaver surgery—a stranger's kidney, greater risks. Then Lily reversed herself again. "She said, 'I want you to have what you want, and that's my kidney. I want to do it for you,' " says Molly now, expecting surgery in about three months. She thinks excitedly of two former patients from KDU, both of whom received sibling transplants a few months ago. "They're doing great, just *great!*" she grins.

But many renal failure patients have no sibling—or a sibling in poor health, who is a poor match, or who simply refuses. Parents and children also can donate, but the risks are higher and the matches poorer. These patients have no choice but a cadaver donor, and they must apply to the program—passing the criteria—and line up for the handouts, for someone to die, waiting sometimes for years. Cadavers are also matched for tissue type, and patients with unusual types wait the longest; they sometimes die waiting. More than one researcher has proposed that a rare tissue type is, like age or disease, an objective criterion on which to refuse a transplant.

Not just any dead stranger will do. He or she should be not too old and not too sick and free of infection and major problems such as drug-controlled hypertension and cancer. There is no better stranger to get your kidney from than a healthy, active young person who has had the bad luck to go through a car's windshield or dive off the shore into a rock—and the good luck to do so close enough to a hospital to be put on a ventilator right away.

S UCH A PERSON, A TWENTY-TWO-YEAR-OLD WOMAN, WAS killed in a head-on collision in Harriet Mercer's "procurement" area recently. Within hours her corneas, the bones of her middle ear, several pieces of cartilage, and both kidneys were removed. The kidneys, matching no one in the area, were flown 1000 miles to another transplant center, pulsing slightly in a machine and flooded with solution. I was sitting with Deb in her sunlit office the following day, talking with her in a languid way about this woman and her requisite parts, when the phone rang. It was the woman's mother, calling from the lobby of the hospital, crying for the first time since the accident. Harriet's voice immediately dropped half an octave and became soothing, caramel, that singsong comfort that seems to work so well with the grieved. The woman's mother wanted to remove her daughter's body for burial in another state, and in the frenzy of organ removal and permission slips, no one had explained to her how this could be done. Standing at a pay phone in the lobby, she wasn't even sure where the body was.

The kind of person whose brain is dead but whose heart beats is fondly known as a "heart-beating cadaver." Every intensive care nurse has taken care of one or more. Aaron was a heart-beating cadaver, but the poison of his meningitis disqualified him as a donor. It is another of the self-created dilemmas of medical technology, another of the active choices. Hard enough to get the phone call, the visit, announcing the sudden and violent death of a husband or daughter. Harder, in its way, to watch the body breathe, see the blip on the monitor go bouncing on its way, to sign the consent forms and say goodbye not to a corpse but to a warm, soft, almost sleeping body, breathing in, breathing out.

Oregon is one of a number of states recently to embrace a new method for dealing with organ donations. In the past a person who died in such a way as to "qualify" as a donor needed either to have carried a donor card—thus encouraging the physicians to approach the family, who still must give permission—or have interested relatives. Many physicians and nurses are reluctant to ask grieving family members (whose relative has so often died suddenly) to discuss organ donation. It is an uncomfortable question to ask, for all the good intentions. So my state recently passed a law to *require* hospital administrators to ask relatives for permission. The reasoning, as I understand it, is if the administrators (who will pass the duty to the physician, nurse, and social worker) are obliged by law to ask an uncomfortable question, they can shift the blame for the discomfort onto the law—and perhaps get a kidney or two in the bargain.

This law is only a step or two behind the idea of "implied consent," in which the law assumes that people want to donate any and all organs unless they carry a card that says they *don't*. If a few things are removed inadvertently before religious or personal objections are lodged by the family, well, so be it. It's the law.

GEORGE, AGE FORTY-FOUR, HAD BEEN ON DIALYSIS ONLY a few months when he was given the kidney of a fourteen-year-old boy who had died in a car accident. The tissue match was so good that the kidney was flown across six states for him. The new organ worked only four days before George's body frantically sent him into rejection, and it was surgically removed.

Of his original illness, George says only, "It had a big name to it." For some reason—he doesn't care what the reasons are—George's own kidneys, never removed, began working again, working just enough to keep him off the machine. He stayed off for two years.

"I thought, 'There we go again,' and I really didn't want to go back," he remembers about the gradual return of symptoms. He refused to return to KDU for six months, until his health declined to the point of incapacitation. He sits now in a big armchair, watching the television, eating french fries. George is a salt-waster, one of the few, and he has no sodium restriction. A fake Russian fur hat covers his thin hair, and he speaks slowly, flatly, with little change of expression as he talks about his experiences. "Hereabout three or four months ago I came as close to death as I'm gonna come. In the back of my mind I thought, 'This is it, I really am dying.'" George knows more than one person who has given up dialysis to die, and he admits that he's considered the possibility. But he shakes his head. "I've always believed that to take my own life was a sin." He is once again on the waiting list.

Dialysis patients can experience something known as the "holiday phenomenon." Patients waiting for cadaver kidneys become elated and relaxed in the days before a three-day weekend. They are waiting for the inevitable increase in traffic deaths, for the healthy person to go through a windshield. If no kidney is offered, depression takes the place of elation. F. Patrick McKegney says, "It's the 'Christmas eve, no Christmas morning,' syndrome in which you go to bed at night thinking you may get a call that night to come in for a transplant, but every morning you wake up, you realize that the phone didn't ring."

George has a sister, and she offered him her kidney as soon as he got sick. But again he shakes his head: "She's the only family I got. If my sister did give me one of her kidneys, then later on something might happen to her— I didn't want that responsibility." He looks at the blood running through the tube out of his arm. "I didn't want her to have to go through this."

Life after transplant, no matter how successful the operation, is not wholly normal either. As the saying goes, sometimes the patient dies. An extraordinary number of side effects follow kidney transplantation, from an inexplicable outbreak of warts over the whole body to a recurrence of the original disease in the new kidney. Five percent of all patients have one or more complications specific to the kidney and bladder, another 10 to 15 percent suffer ulcers, more than half have a variety of eye troubles, and as many as 83 percent—depending on whose research you read—have high blood pressure, which can, and does, cause kidney damage. The new kidney can hemorrhage or rupture, and always the body snarls on its immunological chain to tear it apart.

Except in the very few perfect, identical-twin matches, the body always perceives the kidney as foreign, and rejection is held at bay with drugs, the original parallel course. Steroids are the cornerstone.

T WO TYPES OF STEROIDS, CORTICOSTEROIDS (OF WHICH there are two types, mineral corticoids and glucocorticoids) and androgens, are made by the body from cholesterol. Androgens are the steroids used by bodybuilders and some athletes to increase muscle mass; they have their own set of dangers, mostly disruptions of sexual characteristics. It is the corticosteroids that can muzzle the snarling dog.

In normal physiology, these compounds have extremely complex and varied effects on the body, including essential steps in the metabolism of many nutrients, the balance of fluids and electrolytes (such a delicate tightrope), and the strength of muscle contraction. Many pages would be required even to begin praising the steroids for their role in health, in keeping our bodies calm and alert under stress, our blood properly mixed, and our brains percolating along. Physicians prescribe steroids for a great divergence of problems, from arthritis to asthma. They are very strong anti-inflammatories, controlling and reducing the swelling and pain, not only of arthritis, but also of similar reactions, such as allergic dermatitis and lupus. Steroids are used, obviously, as physiologic replacements in people whose own bodies make too little and to control various intestinal, eye, liver, and skin diseases. Steroids reduce swelling in the brain, ease the danger of shock, make hayfever a little easier to live with. Steroids are commonly used with cancer, because one of the most dramatic effects they have on the body is to depress—that is, slow, quiet, muzzle—the immune system, which can in turn slow the growth of a tumor. Here is where the kidneys come in.

Often the donors, alive or dead, are treated with steroids before surgery. Even before recipients have a new kidney, they are treated with steroids for the rest of their lives. The body never remembers that the kidney belongs there; steroids tie its hands, so to speak, handcuffing the healthy immune response so that it can't fight. At the first sign of rejection, the dose may be increased—up to a point, because steroids can be killers.

The great risk with depressed immunity is, of course, infection. Four out of ten kidney transplant patients die of an infection—pneumonia, bladder infections, blood infections, tuberculosis, viral diseases, Legionnaires' disease. Many of the antibiotics useful in treating such infections cause kidney damage. Steroids cause osteoporosis, a debilitating weakness of bone often seen in the elderly. Both kidney failure and the transplant cause similar weaknesses; the combination can break hips with a slight jolt. Steroids cause diabetes, cataracts, and ulcers; they can inflame the pancreas, damage the liver, and depress the emotions. Steroids also contribute directly to hypertension—high blood pressure—which can cause kidney damage. My most detailed drug reference book lists thirty-nine serious side effects for one brand of steroid alone. People on long-term therapy often develop something called Cushing's syndrome: the face swells and flushes until it is as round and full as the harvest moon; the abdomen grows fat, flabby, stretch-marked and pendulous; and the body grows hair in unexpected places— cheeks, back, and breasts. Cushing's syndrome can only be treated by lowering the dose—risking rejection—but untreated it can lead to confusion, depression, and personality changes.

Posttransplant patients have a greatly increased risk of cancer, probably due to the steroids. Overall, matched for age to the general population, cancers are 100 times more common. A leukemia-like cancer, reticulum cell sarcoma, has an incidence 350 times higher in people who have received a transplant.

C YCLOSPORIN A IS A DRUG ORIGINALLY NOTED FOR ITS antifungal properties. In the past several years it has caused a stir with transplant specialists because it is also a very powerful immunosuppressive. "It's a really tricky drug to manage," says Deb Prewit. Her team gives (cyclosporine A) and prednisone, a steroid, as the first-choice treatment, but many people can't take cyclosporine. Its major side effect is kidney damage. Even though it has almost no other difficulties, this particularly ironic one is the one that matters the most. Prewit's team has used it only a year, and she won't predict the results, although the vague outlook so far is positive.

Baby Fae received steroids and cyclosporine to prevent rejection of the baboon heart she was given in October of 1984. Because Baby Fae was under a kind of stress few humans experience, because her entire life was spent ill and dying, specific blame for specific problems is hard to pinpoint. Clearly, she could never have lived long with a baboon heart; adults who receive human heart transplants often don't live long with the most extensive steroid therapy—although some live years. But they live with Cushing's syndrome and high blood pressure, and Baby Fae could not have survived any of the many blows of rejection—or antirejection treatment. Before her death, Baby Fae's kidneys quit—thanks, perhaps, to the cyclosporine—and for days she, like so many others, was dialyzed.

In all children, steroids can retard growth severely; in some cases they retard mental development and prevent sexual maturation, as well as causing the other side effects. One of the intimate dilemmas of kidney transplantation has been whether to give organ transplants to children, knowing full well what they face afterward. If the transplant is successful (and how do we measure success in this art?), they may be, as one doctor put it, "preadolescent forever."

A number of transplant centers are experimenting with something called OKT3, a monoclonal antibody. Monoclonals are complex substances derived in the laboratory after a series of animal and culture growth steps, and they are full of a kind of promise. Monoclonals are far more specific than such drugs as steroids, aiming at, in the case of OKT3, the T-lymphocyte cells that cause acute rejection. It is an expensive, exceedingly detailed technique, and years will pass before it is either readily available or surely safe.

But safe is a relative word in this netherland. Mercer's team, and others, have returned to an old-fashioned trick for suppressing the immune system before a transplant. In an age of radiation nightmares, they are giving some

patients total lymph node irradiation prior to surgery—
x-rays, radiation, of the whole body.

Fully 60 to 90 percent of closely matched live donor
kidneys are still working after five years, but less than
2000 live donor surgeries were performed in 1983. After
ten years, just over half the people receiving a cadaver
kidney are alive. People who stick with dialysis have as
good a chance at survival as cadaver kidney recipients.

"We see all sides," says Harriet Mercer. She remembers
a young woman who still visits the outpatient clinic. She
had always wanted a baby, but her renal failure clearly
prohibited it. After a transplant, she became pregnant—
"A little sooner than we would have liked," smiles
Mercer—and now she is the mother of a healthy two-
and-a-half-year-old boy. Her kidney is still in fine working
order. "That," Mercer concludes, "makes it all worthwhile."

I N 1972, PUBLIC LAW 92-603, CALLED THE SOCIAL SECU-
rity amendment of 1972, was passed by Congress. Section 2991 extended Medicare coverage to people with
permanent kidney failure. In effect, the act creates a group
of people—under sixty-five and without disability—who
are handicapped simply because of kidney failure. In 1983,
the cost of the end-stage renal disease (ESRD) program
was nearly $2 billion and is expected to be $3 billion by
1988. ESRD is 2.4 percent of the budget of the whole
beleaguered Medicare program going to 0.02 percent of
the Medicare population. These figures also count only
the money spent directly on dialysis and transplants, not
on rehabilitation, hospital costs for complications, and so
on. Nor does it include Social Security disability payments

and other forms of welfare extended to the large percentage of CRF patients who can't or won't work. The program began as a generous statement of the right to health care for all and has become far bigger, far more expensive, than anyone had dreamed. The regulations are a morass of exceptions, subheadings, italics, qualifications, and exclusions.

This escalation is responsible for the current push toward cheaper treatments: Self-dialysis, home dialysis, and transplants. A transplant, for instance, costs about $12,000 for the surgery and about $1200 a year afterward for drugs and exams. In-center hemodialysis is currently running about $26,000 a year. But because a lot of patients are unwilling to go through a long training or a hard surgery when the results are so uncertain, incentives are necessary.

The current approach is a set of new ESRD regulations directed at "encouraging" the cheaper alternatives—encouraging by providing financial rewards to those who choose to dialyze at home. As it stands now, Medicare has quit paying the whole bill presented by a center, and the remainder goes to the patient—who typically cannot pay and eventually goes on welfare. The new regulations penalize facilities which don't actively train patients in self-dialysis. Everyone seems to wonder if there *is* a solution to these unending inflations of money and mazes. There seems no alternative to encouraging the poor to take health risks—except lowering profit margins. Martha Orr suggests we direct cost containment "to the provider side of the equation by reducing the allowable profits."

But the "provider side"—physicians and hospitals, equipment companies, and diasol manufacturers—is unlikely to volunteer. Take the vascular surgeon I mentioned earlier, the one who does button surgeries for needle access for those who can afford it. About half his patients are renal failure patients. He's an unhappy man, sharp, acerbic, a man who enjoys jolting people with his extreme opinions and sarcasm. The nurses in the unit tolerate his manner, even trade seemingly friendly barbs with him, and then turn on him with bared teeth when he leaves. He told me that his job isn't any fun anymore, that the days when patients would send thank-you notes and Christmas cards to their doctors are over; he blames this on the welfare system. The ESRD program, he says, has created a population of people who expect to be provided for, who have lost the motivation to provide for themselves. When I asked him about selection criteria—what characteristics should eliminate a person from receiving a transplant—he added to the standard list one more: poverty.

Ah, encouragement. It predicts a return to the halcyon days of selection criteria. But while before most criteria were subjective judgments of personality and conformity, now objective measures of immunity and success rates can be used. One subtype of immune cells, which can be found by a simple skin test, is associated with transplant rejection. One researcher, reporting this, suggested that such a test could select out a proportion of people "unsuitable" for transplantation. If enormous deficits and spending cutbacks revive the selection committees, the committees will be armed with probabilities and projections, statistics and research, with which to weigh the clamoring candidates.

Nurses see the priorities differently. They spend months with the patients, cajoling, reprimanding, coaxing, watching them fail for want of a donor kidney—or watching them return to the machine when a transplant doesn't work. The cost of one button surgery would pay almost two months of a dialysis nurse's salary. The nurses are spenders, liberals, unhesitant, and unrepentant when it comes to government allocations for their patients. On top of their fear that ESRD cuts and regulations will, in effect, kill some of their patients by long waits and hurried decisions is the anger that they, the nurses, will be forced to carry out the selection. I hear accusations of racism and ageism, that, as one nurse put it, the "criteria's going to be white, male, under sixty—who have insurance to cover part of it." Time after time, nurses compare the cost of various parts of the defense budget—bombs, the MX—to the costs of the ESRD program. To them, entitlement is a correct and precise term: that all of us are entitled to the care available. To cut off the funds is murder.

In California, a young prison inmate serving a term of several years for first-degree burglary receives dialysis treatments three times a week for four hours at a time. He wants to quit: "I'm just walking around on borrowed time. I might as well get it over with." A judge recently ordered the prison staff to continue dialysis over the prisoner's protests, by force if necessary. The law grants equal access, after all.

M ARTHA ORR SPEAKS OF "THE PRINCIPLE OF JUSTICE" in relation to the financial burden of paying for the treatment of kidney failure, of fairly distributing the burden. Justice can be an odd word in the KDU, where unbidden illnesses have wrought such devastation. In a chair down the room from Molly sits a woman in her late twenties, with a clear, plain face. She sleeps curled up in the armchair while her blood is run. Her daughter, eight years old, sits beside her, writing a poem for Molly, who is her friend. This woman has a congenital defect that has destroyed her kidneys. Last year she received a transplant, which appeared successful, but then she developed cancer. When her steroids were withdrawn to slow the cancer, she rejected the kidney, and now she comes again for dialysis as well as treatment for the cancer. On the other side of the room in another chair is her brother. He has the same congenital disease; his kidneys have also failed.

Now and then, dialysis patients do walk away from their treatment and the uncertain future. As a rule, such behavior (called "passive suicide" in the literature) is considered an indication of poor psychological adjustment —hence the prison inmate's strange new sentence. He will be saved; we will save him. He and all his brothers and sisters in the game of blood and waiting are the living monuments of a great society.

I T'S GETTING ON IN THE EVENING NOW; THE NEWS IS OVER and the sitcoms are on. Rain keeps pouring down, but the five hospital floors above the KDU absorb the sound. A few lights have been turned off; a few patients are already on their way home. The voices are drifting farther apart and the intercom is silent. But there's always a steady hum, a Doppler sound that seems to come from a great distance and then recede, again and again, every few seconds. Molly is propped up in the bed in the center of the horseshoe, the bed lifted high and facing the nurses' desk. She is queen of the KDU.

"I have a Living Will," she tells me. "I asked the nurses if they would honor that if something happened to me, and they said no—because I'm young and I'm strong and I have a good heart. They said, 'We wouldn't let you go, we'd try everything we could to keep you.'" Molly is crying now, very quietly, and she seems to shrivel in the high white bed. It is hard to be queen, to keep trying. Molly doesn't see, I suspect, that she *is* the living will—the will of the nurses and doctors, the animation of the inanimate machines. She is the volition, the purpose, the point. Her own life has been bequeathed already. She has beaten death, beaten it by the force of that will. How dare she turn away, ask them to stand idly by? She lives because of that active will.

Ah, mercy. Good intentions. My local newspaper has recently followed the story of a little girl, just two years old, with biliary atresia, a congenital condition of the liver bile ducts that is inevitably fatal. The cry went out for a liver transplant, and the cry went out for money to pay for it. The girl was a ward of the state, living in a foster home, and with enough publicity and testimony, her foster mother was able to get the state legislature to pay for a transplant—$100,000. And a few weeks ago she received one. The liver failed. She received another. She died.

Hearts, lungs, and pancreases, Baby Fae and the artificial heart: every surgery a lesson, every surgery a martyrdom. Some live, some are glad; others live and smile for the cameras, and who knows if Baby Fae was grateful? Life, life above all. Pain is only pain. Each patient is the proof.

"It's always there, always there with you," Molly told me before I left her, before she came off the machine. "You have to take care of yourself because no one else will."

And this, I think, is most troubling of all. Molly has received the best of care, the best we can give her. She has received the exotic, the heroic, the new miracles. Still, she feels neglected. Is she really so spoiled? Or is it just that she feels the trembling machine's heart against her own, beating, beating?

FIRE AND AIR

KIDNEYS DRIP, DRIP; THE TUMOR CELL DIVIDES. THESE are slow and modulated shifts. Their progress is barely visible; we are likely to miss the first signs in our preoccupation. But some adjustments cannot be ignored: they are debacles, physical revolutions. The mind and heart must hurry, struggling, to catch up.

"Some say the world will end in fire," wrote Robert Frost. For some of us, it does. We are drawn to flames, punish with fire, and revel in it. War is fire and so is execution, the pariah strapped into a chair that vibrates with electric flames. Millions are burned to ashes after their death; the Hindu wife is thrown alive on her husband's pyre, her only hope. We burn witches and heretics at the stake, to cleanse them; we dissolve waste, the unwanted, in baths of acid. A mother, driven to distraction by her child's crying, dips him in a tub of scalding water, tosses a cup of coffee in his face.

Fire is both joy and pain—it warms us, cooks our food, grows our crops. "Among all phenomena, it is really the only one to which there can be so definitely attributed the opposing values of good and evil," wrote the philosopher Gaston Bachelard. "If all that changes slowly may be explained by life, all that changes quickly is explained by fire."

A group of recovered burn victims calls itself the Phoenix Society. Each year 2 million Americans are burned; 300,000 are burned seriously. Their unchosen pain becomes a source of teaching: for the unburned to repeat, observe, approve. It is pain as a religious joy, as a religious damnation. Whether the outcome will be ruin or rebirth for any one of these lightning-struck innocents is impossible to predict: destroyed by fire, the past disappears and the future becomes a new world on the other side of the tunnel of the burn unit, through which the victim must crawl all alone.

Relatively few hospitals have specialty burn units. In those that do, the burn unit is the hardest place to enter, the most guarded, the most protected. A friendly surgeon may take a visitor by the hand into the operating room, a class of psychology students may forage through the pediatric floor, but few visitors get into the burn units out of curiosity. In part, this is because of the urgent need to prevent infections, but it is more than that. No casual wanderer would be glad to stumble across the burn unit unawares. Burn treatment is, with rare exceptions, the most extensive treatment medicine offers, and often the most expensive. These uncommon beds start at over $1000 a day, minus the frills. In the burn unit, terrifying and exquisitely painful procedures are done in the name of healing; hideous wounds are repaired as best they can. It is hard to watch, hard to hear, hard to do.

Burn patients are wrapped in white—muted, stilled, suspended. They are attended by people in green and

yellow suits, hair caps, shoe covers, masks, indistinguish-
able by sex or intention. The two societies mingle in an
exclusive club, a family of initiates, a world removed.
There is a muffled quality to the machine sounds—the
whoosh of ventilators, the beep of monitors—broken by
moans, words, the hush of double doors sighing open
and closed, an occasional cry or scream. And unlike the
creeping cataract or growing tumor, burns appear suddenly, abruptly, without warning. The injury becomes a
crucible, and the burn unit becomes a proving ground.

A MAJOR BURN IS POSSIBLY THE WORST THING THAT CAN
happen to a person's body, the worst of all physiologic catastrophes up to the point of death. The treatment
is fraught with oddities. Our skin protects us from infection and ultraviolet rays, helps to balance bodily fluids,
and provides much information about our environment.
Without skin, the human body becomes frenzied and confused. Without skin, the fluids mix and shift, fleeing vital
organs and then filling them, changing blood pressures
and chemical compositions rapidly and disastrously. A
large burn can evaporate almost 3 liters of water every
day. Burns "bleed white," draining precious quantities of
salts, proteins, and nutrients. Untreated, a person with
major burns will die of shock in a few hours. In the desperate metabolic rush to stop the steady flow of fluid out
and the tide of shifting waves within, the body becomes
catabolic, eating its own protein mass. Even after weeks
of seeming stability, a person can suddenly sour and die.

Loss of skin is more than a physical disaster. It is the
loss of our point of contact with each other and the world,
with our shape and form, our view of ourselves—and
others' view of us. Burns remove the borders we use to

take up space, define our shape, push air out of the way. The helplessness that follows goes beyond the extraordinary dependence on nurses, doctors, and machines; it is a helplessness of spirit, of self, identity; it is like a death.

The first hours of a burned person's new life are taken up by "resuscitation," the clearing of pathways for air, the focused beating of the heart. Then the team of physicians and nurses settles into a complex routine of care, which will often last for months. The hole in the body must be plugged, or else we drain away. In the days after the injury, the dead skin and muscle shrink and the tissues swell with fluid, and if a limb is surrounded by burn, its entire blood flow can be squeezed shut. They call this "circulatory embarrassment." Then the burn must be sliced open down its length, like splitting a hot dog before cooking so it doesn't bubble and burst. A chest embraced in this way by dead tissue—called "eschar"—may be sliced with an H or other design, like Zorro cutting his enemy's silken shirts. These cuts don't bleed very much, don't hurt much; there's too little left of blood vessels and pain fibers. This shrinking, too, can pull up joints short and tight, ending motion, making seams and seals where there were none before; between chin and chest, between lips, between eyelids.

Severely burned people have a metabolic need beyond that of ordinary people. Without aggressive nutritional support, the person drops pounds in hours. A not uncommon requirement is 5000 calories a day and many liters of water, carefully balanced and calculated. This is many times the average adult's needs, enough to kill a healthy person if he or she could gag so much food down. Where to put the needle for an IV, the tube down the throat to the stomach, when skin, muscle, and blood vessels are charred away? With the best of care, the nutrition can be inadequate, despite odd mixes of fats and amino acids that taste like syrupy chalk and pour out sluggishly like thick glue.

The burned person is a greenhouse for bacteria, a ready source of dead meat and fresh blood, immobile and compromised. Opportunistic bugs find their way sooner or later into the most controlled units, and that's trouble. Then skin grafts slough off, lungs fill with fluid, bowels run with diarrhea. Antibiotics can kill here, too. In the first hours of shock from the twisting rivers of blood and tissue fluid, the internal organs can be damaged as their oxygen supplies are cut off in the rush. Kidneys are particularly sensitive, and with a damaged kidney, prescribing drugs becomes a tricky procedure indeed. Every manifestation must be deftly parried, like unexpected obstacles appearing on a desperate course. And before long comes the pain, like a sudden Arctic wind on an August day, knocking you over, leaving you breathless and scared.

T WIN BOYS, FIFTEEN MONTHS OLD, AND THEIR FATHER, who pulled them from a burning house. A young pianist, his dominant hand destroyed by flaming oil. A sixteen-year-old girl roasted when a church barbeque exploded, killing her boyfriend. An infant with a scalded face. A forty-four-year-old woman who drank Drano, her mouth a swollen black doughnut. A young man trembling in bed, incoherent, who soaked himself in kerosene and blew himself up. A housewife who spilled a deep fat fryer and slipped in the grease, falling into the puddle and lying there, unable to rise because of an injured back. A two-year-old boy burned in the house fire that killed his mother. A thirty-year-old woman pulled from a burning house, who weeps for her lost face. This is heartbreak, this is tragedy without a shred of sentimentality, without room for romance or morals or poetry, no room for anything but a speechless wonder. Like the lost, dead love of Galatea, "I rage, I melt, I burn. . . ."

Jered, one of the twins, is almost dead. He arrived with 67 percent of his body burned, most of it "full-thickness"—what used to be called third degree. The skin, fat, muscles, blood vessels, and nerves are all destroyed in a full-thickness burn, cooked like the white of an egg. Such burns, with the nerves gone, are curiously painless. Jered had the imprint of a baby blanket on his forehead, the ribbed pattern burned into his scalp, and his airway was filled with soot. He may have been poisoned by the nylon fumes of the burning blanket. His brother Michael is burned almost as deeply, but Michael's lungs are almost clear, so he has a much better chance at survival.

Jered is doped with morphine and Valium to keep him from fighting the ventilator that breathes for him. "I think we're going to get them both well," says the medical director, a surgeon, "but it's going to be a case of zero mistakes."

A curious fact of house fire burns is that one need not be touched by the flames to be so badly hurt. Jered and Michael were pulled from a bedroom not yet burning. Houses on fire grow extraordinarily hot in a few short minutes—1200 degrees, 1500 degrees Fahrenheit—and the skin chars and crisps away as though it were in a kiln. Our homes, our most precious belongings, are the worst kinds of poisons: upholstered chairs, paint, rugs, mattresses all smolder with toxic fumes that can mix with the water in the lungs to form acids—simple acids that burn from the inside out.

In a room separate from both his brother and father —to prevent infections—Michael is awake, angry, and bewildered. All was well a few days ago. Whence came this sudden change? He mews and whines in his crib, face buried in the sheets and diapered bottom high in the air, trying to escape his restraints. He is being fed by an IV in his ankle and a tube down his nose into his stomach, and his toddler scrambling could easily dislodge the precious tubes. Therefore, he is bound to the bars of the crib. He waves his thickly padded arms and tries to struggle with the nurse who comes to turn him. Twice a day his dressings are changed—in the tank.

The tank is the dungeon, the bright, tiled room of dread. Michael's nurse Linda tells me about a recent patient, a middle-aged woman. "She couldn't sleep at night because she dreaded the tank. The first thing she'd say to me in the morning was, 'Let's get it over with.' It was terribly painful for her. Then she'd spend the rest of the day thinking about how many hours until her next tanking. When I'd bring her pain medication to her, she'd say, 'Oh, now it's only thirty minutes until I go in the tank!' "

The tank is out of vogue in some places now, but it is standard procedure at this particular unit, one of the largest and most respected in the country. Almost every patient here will be tanked for at least part of his or her stay, some twice daily for many weeks.

The tank or tub is often a stainless steel table with high sides and drains, not unlike the tables used for autopsies. Other tubs are like giant shiny spas, many feet wide and long and deep enough to soak in. The patient is either scrubbed and showered with a nozzle or soaked in water, to help peel off dressings, wash off medicine, and soften the dead skin, which must be cut or shaved off. Patients are immediately tanked when they arrive from the ambulance, to clean the wounds and protect against infection. It is often the nurses' job, when they bathe, to take forceps and knives or scissors and pull up patches of dead skin and muscle, clipping until the wound is clean. A full-thickness burn is painless, but when the edges begin, ever so slightly, to heal, the fresh new pain fibers are electrically sensitive when exposed to air, washed, touched, scrubbed. All partial-thickness burns—first and second degree—are exquisitely painful from the beginning. Remember grabbing the pan without a pot holder, pulling back in pain before the realization is conscious? Remember the angry red, the blister? Imagine two-thirds of your body.

Even with burns covering 95 percent of the body, people are often lucid when admitted to the hospital, some even euphoric before lapsing into unconsciousness. Patients don't realize how badly they are injured because at first there is no pain. All the fuss seems unnecessary, overwrought, a bit silly. But with time a dream state of dissociation begins, separate from the experience, and it can be either a happy fantasy or a repetitive nightmare in which the crisis is relived again and again. Some recovered patients cannot remember the first few weeks of treatment and critical care. Pain without memory. Is it real?

TIME FOR MICHAEL TO GO IN THE TANK. HE IS CARRIED into the room fully bandaged. I wheel his IV pole behind. Three nurses gather round the tub, masked and gowned with sterile gloves on, as though in surgery. Using scissors, one nurse begins to cut away the thick gauze around his chest while another unwinds the roll around his leg. I can't tell who is who; I open packages when supplies run out, hold a bandage so it won't unfurl. As his dressings come off, Michael begins to roll from side to side, struggling to get his hands and knees, away. All three nurses work to hold him still. As each limb is exposed, the skin is scrubbed with antiseptic soap and showered, two and three times, and patches of dead skin are clipped off. I try to stroke his head, greasy with ointment and sweat, and he seems unaware of the attention. I feel shocked, cold, like a victim of unexplained violence. His hands, his feet, his face are all badly burned. He wiggles and cries in a steady ululation, alien, growling through a smoke-sore throat.

Once the wounds are clean, the nurses slather a white antibiotic cream called Silvadene in thick coats all over his body, wrap whole rolls of soft gauze around each area, and then cover his legs, arms, and trunk with mesh gauze, a highly elastic cotton tubing that can be cut and shaped like clothing to hold the dressings in place. Each finger and toe is painstakingly separated and wrapped singly. Ties cut off surgical masks are used to bind the Stockinette pieces together until, almost an hour after beginning, Michael is clothed from head to toe in a thick, mesh-white bodysuit with small holes for his eyes and mouth. He waves his arms, padded oars, helplessly. I ask Linda how long before his next tubbing. She laughs: "You're just like my patients! Don't dwell on it." In eight hours the process will begin again.

Now Linda holds him. She sits in a wooden rocking chair around the corner from the open door, with the lights down low, and pulls the bound boy up against her uniform. She whispers to him through her mask. Linda is trying to get pregnant and is afraid she might be infertile. Michael quiets, stills his movements, and presses his face tight in between her breast and the arm which encircles him.

A FULL-THICKNESS BURN OF 1 INCH DIAMETER WILL TAKE over three months to heal spontaneously. Because of these exceedingly long periods, all full-thickness burns and many partial-thickness burns are closed surgically. One method, especially for smaller burns, is called "excision and closure." In surgery, the entire burn is excised—cut out—and then neighboring skin is pulled over to close the wound much as a regular surgical wound is closed. There is the chance for considerable loss of blood in such a procedure. Most large-area burns are closed with grafts, to plug the hole through which life drains away.

Grafts take three forms: xenografts, from another species (almost always pigskin); hemografts, from cadavers; and isografts, the patient's own skin. There is an odd exception: Someone who has had a bone marrow transplant in the past may develop an immunity against his or her own skin and only be able to accept the bone marrow donor's skin as his or her own. The search for a good artificial skin has failed so far; nothing shares the porosity and elasticity of human skin.

Pigskin is cheap, considering; a patch about 3 inches by 4 inches costs around $13. The skin is harvested in the slaughterhouse and bought by hospitals in sealed packages, frozen or dried. The same size patch of cadaver skin costs $59, because there isn't as much to go around. Organ donors don't usually think about skin when they agree to donate their own or a dead relative's body parts, and they often refuse when specifically asked for skin. The idea causes disquiet somehow. A skin bank technician tells me that this is why they always try to get blanket consents for *any* organ.

His is a specialized job. He is in charge of removing the skin from dead bodies once permission is obtained, a procedure called harvesting. It must be done within hours of death, twenty-four at the most if the body has been refrigerated. He and his assistants will travel hundreds of miles on little or no notice to harvest. He keeps the skin in a heavy square freezer in a corner of his office, stored in liquid nitrogen at extremely low temperatures. You handle this smoking material carefully, with gloves: it burns.

A person borrows the skin of others only briefly. The body rejects it the same as if you tried to sew a gauze bandage on and call it fur. No one's fooled. Pigskin and cadaver grafts will stay in place several days, covering the wound until the cells begin to regenerate (in a partial-thickness wound) or a victim's own skin can be harvested for a permanent graft.

You go to your grafting surgery a sheep to the fleecing. The skin is removed, delicately, with instruments called dermatomes and dermabraders. Manual or electric, large or small, they are like souped-up cheese slicers. Gloved hands slide the knives along and peel the skin off in fine transparent sheets. Split-thickness grafts, most common, are simply the fragile top layer. Deep split-thickness and full-thickness grafts are thicker chunks with better blood supplies, promising better cosmetic results for faces and hands. Oh, those anatomic apportionments of the skin we hold so dear.

Weeks from now, when the sites are healed, they may be stripped again—and even again. Almost any part of the body can be used, including the scalp. (To graft an eyebrow, of course, one goes first to the scalp and its hair follicles.) If only a little unburned skin remains, the graft can be turned into mesh in a machine called a skin-ex-pander, stretched to a great size, and laid along the wound like a net stocking. New skin grows between the wicker-work; it forms scars of lace.

N ANCY IS THIRTY YEARS OLD; SHE TURNED THIRTY JUST last week. She is a smoker—strike one. She has bronchitis—strike two. And the night her house caught fire, she'd taken antihistamines to help her sleep and was too sedated to escape. Her boyfriend pulled her from the fire. Her arms, thighs, and face were burned; her lungs were damaged by smoke.

"It's the north breeze," she complains about the cold oxygen blowing down her throat from the mask, in a gravelly, strained whisper. "My throat hurts so much." Nancy has had both arms grafted with meshed skin from her calves, filigree, and her arms hover out in front of her like the limbs of a tree, wrapped and padded. The dressings will stay on the grafts for several days to prevent any disturbance of the delicate new connections. But her other burns and her graft donor sites must still be cleaned and rebandaged.

The most obvious problem with skin grafting is that donor sites scar, much like burns, but in the symmetrical and geometric patterns taken by the dermatomes. Donor sites are very painful, much like a fresh minor burn, and they sting, itch, and bleed freely. Nancy's legs tremble as I hold them for the dressing change, bright red blood pours from the pearly wounds. "Can't you give me something for the pain? Can't you give me something to knock me out?" Nancy has already been given her medication; she must endure. Across her shoulders, under one arm, and up to curl around a soft breast is an elaborate and colorful tattoo, a dragon wrapped around a flowering tree, his teeth bared at her nipple. I have a small tattoo on one shoulder, and several years later I still remember the moments of multiplied bee stings that made it. I can imagine what this elaborate mural has cost Nancy in freely chosen pain, a smiling grimace, gritted teeth for a defiant work of art. I compliment her on her dragon, but she is, at the moment, not interested.

Mesh grafts, if they work, form scars exactly as though a windowscreen had been pressed firmly against the area, crocodile skin, a ridged pattern of diamonds. Grafts often fail. Nancy's neighbor is a two-year-old boy whose mother died in the house fire that burned him. He breathed so much smoke that his brain and optic nerves were damaged from lack of oxygen. He is blind, almost mute, rigid when held, and crying when left alone. He is on his third set of grafts; the first two became infected—part of the problem with burns near the buttocks and genitals, especially in a child wearing diapers. Very rarely does a person with extensive burns have a perfect "take" of a set of grafts, because the capillaries must grow into the area within hours for it to heal. The process is repeated as often as necessary until every open area is healed.

Fingers are difficult to graft, because of their shape and the need to keep each mobile. Tiny fingers like Michael's pose the additional problem of growing bones, which push against slowly healing grafts. Between fingers and toes grow blankets of tight red skin that weld joints together, even with the most diligent of care.

Another option, less commonly used, is the tube pedicle, wherein a flap of skin is almost completely removed with its blood supply, twisted on one final thread, and attached to a difficult-to-graft area, where it grows between its original home and the wound. A tube might run from the top of the shoulder around to a destroyed nose, a tube of healthy skin growing to cover the nose until the repair is complete. In this manner hands are attached to chests, arms to chins. For weeks patients walk around splinted to themselves.

To slow down the tightening tendons, several treatments are used. Active range-of-motion exercises are universal and imperative: simply to move the joints the ways they are intended to move. This is not as easy as it sounds. Several times a day a physical therapist or nurse will sidle up to the bedside and, against pain, resistance, and stiffness, bend fingers, toes, wrists, elbows. Bend and stretch. The enforced motion is essential, because patients will encourage the shortened joints by their pain postures—the way they hold themselves to reduce discomfort. Pain postures are always the shortest line between two hinged bones, and the line gets shorter every day.

Another method is traction and forced positioning. Tiny pins are drilled or glued into the fingernails and the hand hung by these pins from a rack. Pins can be inserted in ankles, wrists, even chins to hold a joint in a certain position. The devices used to string up a joint have been named banjos, hayrakes, and halos for their shapes. To keep chin and chest from welding together, a person with neck burns may lie with head hyperextended for weeks, looking at the juncture of wall and ceiling. After traction comes the splints, worn all day and night and removed only for range-of-motion exercises.

Without such management, the results are poor indeed. "Claw hands" are one possibility: hands reduced almost to stumps, fingers only short lumps at the end of a fixated, inflexible limb. A surgeon told me about a woman whose hand was so badly burned that the doctors wanted to amputate and give her an artificial limb. She refused, and instead spent weeks with her hand embedded in a pedicle in her belly. She now has a flipper, fat and stiff and useless—thalidomide hand. "We still see her in the clinic sometimes," he said. "She cries every time." He shook his head, unable to understand why she still refuses the amputation.

"I NEVER GET BORED," LINDA TELLS ME. "WHAT I GET tired of is causing pain." But the pain—that is the point.

Luke is a twenty-five-year-old man who tried to kill himself three weeks ago. He removed all his clothes, poured kerosene over his body, and ignited it. The explosion must have been glorious. He came to the burn unit with 65 percent of his body burned, almost all of it full-thickness. This is at the edge of what is called "unprecedented survival." Because Luke is young and otherwise healthy and because his lungs were only slightly injured, he has a chance. He arrived coherent enough to say that he had tried to kill himself, and since then he has been almost completely nonverbal, apparently delirious. The first paper in his already thick chart is a detailed discussion of the state law allowing medical care for "incompetent" adults.

Most of the damage was done to his legs, although his arms, trunk, face, scalp, neck, and genitals are burned too. He does not go to the tank; he is bandaged in bed by a team of three nurses, who start with his legs. The dressings unroll, and already he is rising off the bed as best he can, teeth bared, staring at the nurses. He growls and grunts. Luke's legs are shredded and bloody, the feet a shiny black, the shins showing bare bones. As his thighs are washed, he lifts, trembling, off the bed as though an electric shock is running through him, back arched and lips drawn back in a grimace.

Pain is the sacrament of burn care, the expectation, essential, unavoidable. Patients are given narcotics in the half-hour before dressing changes, but they serve only to dull—to dissociate—the pain. Combine the drugs, the routine, and the many procedures with the intense pain, and an aura of unreality is created; the patients float, dreaming, losing track of time and day and place. As you stand by the bed or tub you want to stop this pain. You want to do whatever can be done to take it away—give more drugs, stronger drugs, smother the cries with a nearby pillow, knock the moaning child out just so she'll stop. Your helplessness is palpable. Your job is to cause more pain.

One researcher describes it as a "kaleidoscopic experience, a series of discrete, severely painful procedures punctuating the day and night." It has a quality beyond ordinary pain, beyond the ache of a fractured leg or a fresh surgical wound; I think this is so because it carries with it mutilation and mutation, the demand for a new face, a new life. A person is literally unraveled by the pain, rent open, peeled. Burn pain is a leap beyond: "In the realm of suffering, affliction is something apart, specific, and irreducible. It is quite a different thing from simple suffering." When Simone Weil wrote these words, she meant to show the reader a road to God. She is not the first to find in physical pain and psychic suffering a trial and a purpose. To Elaine Scarry, it is "the making and unmaking of the world." Aristotle cautioned us that the wise person looks not for pleasure, but merely for freedom from pain. This is all the burned person begs for; if he or she begs for God, it is only for His intervention. For a life in which he needn't beg for God in pain.

To stand by a bedside and pull the bandages off the wounds, however gently, is to participate in this affliction. But the bandages must be changed. How odd, then, that people who spend their professional lives in burn care cannot agree about the nature—or even the strength—of this pain. When C. S. Lewis lost his wife to cancer, he exhorted a God he was no longer sure he believed in: "Already, month by month and week by week you broke her body on the wheel whilst she still wore it. Is it not yet enough?"

There is a long-standing argument among the researchers. Although all agree that the pain can be excruciating, disagreement remains on how constant and how disrupting the pain is to the patient. To be the perpetuator of frequent intense pain appeals to few of us, and I suspect the elaborate efforts of some writers to downplay the problem is a desire to be free of it, to atone for it. The textbooks themselves devote precious little space to pain: a 1982 burn-care textbook of over 550 pages discusses pain for less than 4 pages, in scattered paragraphs. A study of nurses' attitudes toward burn pain concluded that over half delayed giving narcotics in order to reduce the chances of addiction. Another study, in which both nurses and patients were interviewed, found that the patients claim their pain is worse and their medication less effective than nurses believe it to be.

The writers are particularly careful to remind their peers that what *looks* like pain may in fact be simply anxiety, fear, or depression and that we mustn't be too easily manipulated by the patient. How embarrassing for a physician to discover that her young charge afflicted with third-degree burns of the legs and genitals was merely pulling the wool over her eyes, that he was not really hurting that much, that he could have survived another hour or four without his morphine! Such deception makes a fool out of the doctor and nurse, who have been unnecessarily generous with their goods. After all, anxiety, fear, depression—all these conditions can be treated separately, charted differently, discussed apart. The pain must not be given weight merely because the patient claims it exists, because the patient is under the mistaken impression that he or she may be pain-free, and such is not the case. The search is on for a scientific measurement of pain in order to make it objectively real.

Research is done to prove that pain hurts because so little can be done to relieve it. It is not just a matter of giving more narcotics. Too many narcotics can depress the respiratory system, leading to shallow, ineffective breaths, a problem that becomes very serious for a person with smoke-inhalation damage. Narcotics add to the dreamy, otherworldly quality of the unit and can make fear and anxiety worse by taking away a sense of control. And fear and anxiety *do* increase pain, without a doubt, so their presence is relevant. The desire for an objective measurement and a source of blame stems not just from guilt, but from impotence.

In this light, the casual attitude of the staff takes on a tender side. Dressing changes and tubbings are often accompanied not only by nurturing words and calm explanations, but by conversation between staff about family and personal problems, sports, recipes, troubles with the supervisor or schedule, diets, and the latest group of medical students. Without this detachment, the pain strikes you in the face like a haymaker, like an unexpected splash of cold water. That visceral urge to be rid of it—to *make it go away*—would win out. To stay on the job you have to be able to hold up the trembling leg, hold down the struggling child, and think of other things.

Animals can be made crazy by unpredictable, uncontrollable pain. Researchers call it "experimental neurosis." The concept is well-known to professional torturers: it is not the intensity of the pain alone that breaks a person down—it is not knowing when it will occur, having no way to anticipate, prepare for, or control it, not being able to associate the pain with anything you have done to deserve it. It shatters the defenses.

Learned helplessness is a kind of experimental neurosis in which the person quits fighting and withdraws. It is characterized by "agitation followed by lethargy and depression, feeding disturbances, decreased ability to learn new associations between responses and outcomes, and chronic anxiety. Burn victims are . . . eventually unable to distinguish painful from nonpainful events." In a very real sense, this is only a logical extension of surrender, the rendering up of the identity to the demands of the care givers. Sick people are allowed to deviate, exempt themselves from responsibility, put themselves in the hands of others.

A "successful adjustment" to the role, though, carries

the requirement that the sick person acknowledge that to be sick is bad. Being sick, you must work to overcome it, cooperate with the authorities, agree to return to health if possible. Too much withdrawal, too much surrender, becomes a negative thing—maladjustment. Many burned children begin to withdraw and become passive within a few days of the injury, lapsing into a kind of flaccid unconsciousness when the "painful events" begin. The organism has an instinct for survival, to preserve the fighting energy for a later time, when it may make a difference. The lack of control is everything. Burned children are like rats in cages with electrically impregnated floors who, once they discover that there is no escape when the shocks begin, lie still and quiescent until the shocks are over. Such rats eventually make no attempt to leave even when an exit is offered, but stare at the open door as though it were beyond understanding. No wonder, then, that badly burned children have long-term, sometimes lifelong, psychological troubles.

T HERE IS ANOTHER ELEMENT THAT IS THE PARTICULAR burden of children: abuse. Almost one of every five childhood burns is the result of child abuse. Unlike the slap that sends the child sprawling into the wall, the spontaneous burst of rage or loss of control, most abuse burns are careful and deliberate. Children receive what are called stocking and mitten burns, scalds that extend up the feet to midcalf or up the hands to the wrist from being dipped in boiling water. They have patterns of stove burners and heating grills seared into the skin, polkadots of cigarette burns, coffee splashes like paint on the chest. Most burn-abused children are infants and toddlers, and they are much more likely to die of their injuries than a child burned accidentally, apparently because of their passivity.

Nurses can spot suspicious situations not just from the pattern and type of burns, but from the reaction of the child to pain from the first day: abused children tend to lie there and "take it," unprotesting, instead of screaming and struggling for escape. They have long ago learned that escape is impossible.

One afternoon, gowned like the other nurses and observing the returning patients in the clinic attached to a small burn unit, I watched a burned baby be admitted. I was an extra hand on a busy day; the resident, after a quick exam, turned to me and dropped the crying child in my arms. He was a handsome boy, plump and pink from his howls. Across his chin and neck and chest was an irate red puddle, spilling in drops onto his arms and thighs. Coffee? Cocoa? No one knew. The baby's grandfather, we were told, had brought him to the emergency room moments before, saying the boy had pulled a cup of something hot on top of himself—and then the grandfather, angry, had left. Name, whereabouts of the parents, no one seemed to know. Oh, he cried, this baby, pushing his head in under my arm the way I'd seen Michael do to Linda, seeking escape. We rolled him on a stretcher and wrapped him in gauze, cooing and singsonging to him, leaving the clinic patients to wait in the hall. "What is your name?" everyone called to him, musically as adults do to babies. The head nurse brought a syringe of magenta-colored syrup, laced with codeine, and sip by sip coaxed it down his throat. He finally slept.

For the rest of the afternoon, the nurses' conversation kept returning to abuse. All nurses have a story, a particular child, they remember best. The head nurse is adopting a baby girl who was burned by her natural mother; after the months of care in the unit, she couldn't bear to let her go to a stranger's home. Each, too, remembers children they always suspected of being abused, but for which there was no definitive proof. Perhaps these are the worst. To cause pain is hard; here it is simply what needs to be done. To cause pain because of another's cruel blow, because a person lost control—that is just too much. The anger at abusing parents is marbled with hate, a slow, cool hate. Abused children are repeaters: if returned home (and they often are), the likelihood of another burn injury happening to the same child is 30 to 70 percent.

Somewhere in this trial is a middle way, a balance of pain and compassion. Burn nurses find it or quit. It is a narrow trail flanked by extremity. One side, the side of empathy, is filled with wrenching sorrow, anger, and despair. It is where another person's pain becomes so visible, so inarguably present, that we attempt to take it on as we might carry a burden. This fails because, though we might succeed in weighing ourselves with the burden, we cannot actually take the weight from another: the burden doubles. We have *created* pain. And when we see another's pain (this is not as easy as it may at first seem), we quickly begin to expect the person to behave in certain ways, to respond as we would respond—or are responding—to the same affliction. We make demands of the sufferer, be it patient, child, a whole population. This is the way of the martyr; it is filled first with pity and then with contempt.

On the other side is a kind of total severance from the person in pain. This is more than detachment—it is actually a fissure within the person not in pain from his or her own memory and experience. Because medical science defines pain as physical, the clinician may not only fail to recognize nonphysical experience, but demand that it stop when he does recognize it. This is the World Series of artificial hearts, the unblinking preparation of the heart-beating cadaver. This is the undermedication of the patient in pain, for his own good.

Along the narrow road, where the nurses scrape little

Michael's naked nerves, is a simple acceptance. Here is now, this is happening, keep walking. To project another's experience onto oneself (how would *I* feel; what if this were *my* child?) is both terribly necessary and terribly dangerous. Burn nurses work here year after year, anonymously, cutting off skin and treading lightly. It is easy to slip. They must help each other up when they fall.

S CARS ARE NOT INERT, INANIMATE MATERIAL. THEY ARE alive but dormant, and they can continue to grow and change for years. The healing of a burn wound is complex, a dance of skin cells and connective tissue that varies with every individual. People have a level of "burn resistance," which is thought to have a genetic base and which helps determine how their wounds heal. After the first few days of care, in all but the most critically ill, concern with scars becomes second only to pain—and eventually surpasses it.

Grafted areas almost always appear better than a similar wound allowed to heal by itself. But grafted areas tend to perspire less, produce less oil, itch, and have scattered and sparse hair growth. The new skin, grafted or not, can't be exposed to sunlight for over a year, and for many months it is sensitive to friction and temperature changes, bubbling up with blisters from even a small irritation.

Most grafts are the paper-thin split-thickness type. Full-thickness grafts, used most often on the face, hands, feet, and joints, have another oddity: if taken from an area of the body with more fat deposits, such as the outer thigh or abdomen, the graft can gain weight in its new home as though it had never moved, grow thick and soft and flaccid.

Burned skin changes color. The melanocytes, cells in skin that determine both original color and how much a person will tan, behave erratically and unpredictably as a burn heals. A dark person becomes lighter in spots, a lighter person gets patched with dark areas. (A thin blond woman, splotched, with brown spots leaking out of her clothes.) Makeup is little help. A black nurse who works with burn patients says, "There are no products on the market currently that will work for black skin. People are as disappointed with theatrical paint that looks theatrical as with the burn itself." Makeup of any kind irritates the highly sensitive new skin, clogs already dry pores, and causes rashes and blisters. Surgeons, if they have the leeway, may try to match skin color in a graft, but often there isn't enough skin to worry about such niceties. Some surgeons have even attempted to tattoo grafts to improve the color.

Certain scars have a life and purpose all their own. These are the keloid and hypertrophic scars, fungating and florid tissue that spreads across the line of injury over healthy skin, massive and hard and in high-ribbed ridges across the skin. They are particularly attracted to the face, and blacks are at the highest risk. A young man in the clinic has a back covered with them, running across him like smooth, cooled lava or a groundcover of mushrooms all melded together, hideous. They have a life of their own, apart from the skin around them, from one's wishes, one's dreams. The young man watches me watch him, his eyes brimming, ashamed.

These scars also have a great many—too many—tiny blood vessels, so that they are bright red in color. They can grow and change for many years. This rank and vegetal growth mocks a person long after the wounds are healed, after he or she is pronounced well, even dictating clothing.

A badly burned person wears a new sheath of skin for

life. The skin is like an unwelcome garment, like wool underwear in July. But on top of this goes more: they are called pressure garments, and the metaphor is obvious.

Pressure garments are lightly woven elastic body stockings that reduce the size and stiffness of scars. They are designed to fit particular areas—hands, legs, chests. They are worn twenty-four hours a day, winter and summer, and over time will compress hard, rigid scars to a softer, less garish shape. The stockings are hot. They are restrictive. They are a flag, a sign, another idiosyncrasy of the burned. Over pressure garments may go stiff, broad boots, to shape feet, and the ubiquitous splints for elbows, wrists, shoulders, knees, and necks.

The pressure garments can help with all but the face. Badly scarred faces are in a category of their own.

"Without their faces, human beings could hardly be human at all," writes Norman Bernstein, a psychiatrist and the author of a book devoted to the emotional problems of people with disfigured faces. All our ideals of beauty and ugliness begin with the face. Our ideal of the soul, of the mirror each person can hold for another, of expression and duplicity and the recognition of common experience, begins in the face. People who have lost their faces are not handicapped. They are eunuchs. Others cannot bear to look upon them; if they could, they would be met by a stiff, mummified bed of scars that cannot show emotion. They die a social death, if not a physical one. Said Dante in Hell: "And I, when he stretched out his arm to me / searched his baked features closely, till at last / I traced his image from my memory / in spite of the burnt crust." The neurologist Oliver Sacks, speaking of the similar fate of the Parkinson's disease patient, calls it "ontological outrage."

Masks, not pressure garments, are made to treat facial scars. Technicians who specialize in the work make molds of the person's scarred face and then whittle down the result to an approximation of its former self. A mask is cut from the mold and fitted with straps, and holes are cut for the eyes, nose, and mouth. The masks are either transparent or opaque, as the person wishes; some appreciate the transparency and feel less isolated; others welcome the opaque curtain that hides their mutilation from others. Like the stockings, the masks are worn all day and night for nine months to a year. I almost want to go have a cast thrown for myself, just in case, to ensure the best resemblance if the need arises.

The possibilities are astounding. Synthetic ears and noses, built-up chins and fleshed-out cheeks, transplanted eyebrows and grafted lids all form in the hands of plastic surgeons and their lab technicians. If an eye has been destroyed, an artificial one can be fitted into a reconstructed socket. Lips that are burned badly enough to be excised in surgery can be regrown by a flap of the tongue; several years after such an operation, the tongue is usually mobile and appears normal, and the new lip is only mildly redder and bumpier than its predecessor. Mouths can also be reformed with "mouth expanders," orthodontic appliances gone wild that stretch the lips wide and open. Textbooks show us before-and-after pictures, first the monstrous gap, then the surgeon's skill. The presumably contented model attempting to smile, a bit awkwardly, for the camera. Sometimes the pictures have black slashes across the eyes, as though they had been found in a raid on a pornography store. I find this especially odd: who would recognize these stricken countenances?

A person may put his or her face on in the morning, after it has lain all night on the dresser. The ear and nose and even the eye can be attached to a thick pair of glasses, and it all goes on at once, with a tuck here and there. The prostheses become the person's real face, not a crutch, as much a part of him or her as the skin used to be. The results are unpredictable, but often surprisingly realistic from a distance; even pores and freckles can be created. It can be enough that a person will go to the grocery store, to the bank, for a walk, without too many heads turning, too many children pointing. But if we live somewhere in our bodies—if, like Dr. Sassall, we can't be touched around the eyes—what happens when the eyes are lost? The womb, the source, is violated and the self leaks out.

NORMAN BERNSTEIN TELLS THE STORY OF ROBERT C., who was burned in a car accident at the age of twenty-one. He was a hitchhiker, a soldier going home on leave, and when the car he was riding in crashed into a semi-truck, he was thrown clear of the wreckage. He ran into the flames and pulled the driver out, a hero. The driver died, and Robert was deeply burned on the arms and face. He lost eight fingers, both ears, his nose, his eyelids, and almost all his facial skin and hair. Bernstein shows us a picture of Robert midway through his recovery. He is minimalist, taut. His eyes are too large, too wet, unframed by lids and lashes. The eye globes seem to bulge out of the white face. His nose is two holes, a little bloody. Why go on? Robert seems unfinished, cruelly so, as though God quit making him in a fit of pique. He is rough, accidental, fetal without being smooth.

"Each person who looked at Robert had to make an effort to think of him as a human being. Some children have come up to him when he was sitting in a car and asked 'what he was' and how he came to look that way. While he was visiting a friend's house, a teenage girl walked into the room and saw him. She said what a horrible-looking mask he was wearing and tried to remove it." Robert lives with his parents, who care for him like a toddler because of his lost fingers. He rarely leaves the house, living on the insurance settlement that followed the accident. "As he spoke to me alone he began to talk about the hopelessness of his life and how people always turn to look at him. He said he could bear small children because they said what was on their mind, but adults were "more sneaky" and pretended not to see him, and then turned around and nudged each other." As, I fear, would I.

Robert can't wipe himself after he goes to the bathroom (he has no fingers), can't pull up his pants, button a shirt, or feed himself. An artificial hand has thus far been impractical because of the tenderness of the skin on his arms, "I think there is no good solution to his anxieties," ends Bernstein, sadly. Dante followed Virgil into hell and wept—and Virgil turned on him in contempt. "Still?" he demanded. "Still like the other fools? There is no place for pity here."

GOOD COP, BAD COP. THE TORTURER IS A FRIEND. SUCH problems that the outside world present turn the proving ground of the hospital into home. Some patients hate to leave. They look forward to more surgeries because it is only in the safe shield of the hospital that they feel accepted. Around them are other scarred faces, people who are used to their new faces. Sherry is the sixteen-year-old girl whose boyfriend was killed when a barbeque blew up on them at a church picnic. She has been in the hospital three months, and she would have been discharged earlier except for a puzzling problem with her scalp donor site. The area refuses to heal, and Sherry may not have complete growth of her hair when it has healed. She has been remarkably stoic and determined during her recovery, always cooperative and never shirking exercises or dressing changes. Until now. Now she has begun staying in her room, vomiting frequently, crying. "It's probably time for her to have a good breakdown," says the hospital social worker. "She's been protected here, and soon she'll have to go home."

One day Sherry is walking along the hallway, shuffling in a robe and slippers. She has two prominent front teeth and two gaps from missing teeth in a petite face framed by gauze. Her head, arms, and legs are all encased in either bandages or pressure garments. She smiles at the head nurse and asks, "Please come and see me soon, today. I need to talk to you." When the nurse arrives, Sherry is sitting cross-legged on her bed, surrounded by posters, flowers, stuffed animals, a radio, and a pile of magazines. She has questions about her skin, questions she has been steeling herself to ask.

The nurse knows what to do; she pulls a chair up close and takes Sherry by the hand and touches her all the while they are talking. She strokes the scars on her arms and fingers, pulls down her mitten to look at her palm, rubbing, tapping, and caressing the skin. Sherry lost a thumb on one hand. She explains how the scars will continue to change and eventually look less threatening than they do now, still so early. "So," she concludes, repeating for the fourth time what Sherry desperately wants to hear, "you know that the scars will be less rigid"—she strokes a stiff line that runs the length of a forearm—"less red"—she taps a red palm—"and less dry. Less rigid, less red, less dry." No promises of beauty here, but a tough and loving honesty—and acceptance. Here is a nurse to admire.

Bernstein talked to nurses, physicians, social workers, and psychologists who work with burned people. None felt wholly capable of coping with disfigured people; all felt helplessness and pity. The medical personnel couldn't turn to the mental health specialists for help because the main reaction of many mental health workers is one of unqualified horror. Certainly it is work you either become used to or quit—but if a person doesn't leave burn care within a few months of starting, he or she may stay for many years, may in fact find it almost impossible to leave. This is partly like the nurses in dialysis, who thrive on the technical challenge and relish the demands of critically ill people—where can you go after this? Everything is downhill from here. I meet nurses who have worked in burn care five years, eight years, even ten years. The most successful are the ones who can take a day and work in a clinic, or with minor burns, and get away from the severely injured people. Nurses grow dependent on each other in such a place, knowing that if they or their peers reach the end of a rope, someone will catch them, recognize the signs, take them away. "There is a tendency to become compulsive when caring for severely burned individuals," writes a nurse. One unit calls their tradition of going out for drinks "burn beers."

"WITH A CHILD WE WOULD NEVER QUIT. WITH AN adult—maybe, only if there was no hope of survival, no chance," a burn specialist tells me, standing in the door of Jered's room, where he still lies unconscious on a ventilator. Jered's lungs have suddenly filled with fluid; his blood pressure is erratic. The doctor means never, no matter the prospects. Such is the nature of technology: it sets a standard, a constantly escalating standard that must be met. Once started, it is very hard to stop. No one wants to pull a plug alone, be the judge, take the risk. There is always the slight possibility that one is wrong, and even more of a possibility that someone will claim you are.

Much has been written about the zealousness of doctors, their secret and public motivation not to quit. I know I have a different morality from these doctors—and that they see me as the odd one out. But I don't think, in the end, that my motivations and theirs are all that polar. We want to see less suffering in the world—that is all. Where we part ways is just how much a kind of suffering death would be, to such a child as Jered, to countless other sick and dying people in hospitals around the country. Here we part as nurse and physician, as women and men, as more. It is a greater pain, to me, to watch the ventilator breathe than to wash the body. Is it to Jered?

In 1977, a nurse and physician published an unusual article in the *New England Journal of Medicine*. The authors revealed that in their burn center they had gradually adopted a policy of "autonomy" for burn patients so badly injured that survival was unprecedented, either because of age or the degree of burn or both. In such cases, the entire burn team enters the patient's room while the physician explains the situation. "The presence of the burn team serves to witness and validate the patient's desires and requests, gives consensus to the gravity of the situation, and supports the physician member of the team in this delicate, painful task." While the patient is still lucid, the doctor explains that death must be expected whether or not treatment is intensely given. "At this point, those who interpret the diagnosis of a burn without precedent of survival as an indication to avoid heroic measures typically become quite peaceful." Of the adults admitted to this unit in the two years preceding the article, twenty-four were given this choice. Twenty-one chose to forego treatment, and all twenty-four died.

The hours that follow involve comfort care alone. Pain is controlled as much as possible, but complete sedation is avoided. No ventilators are used, so the patients can speak. No antibiotics, supplemental feedings, or surgery is begun, oxygen is given only to relieve discomfort, and dressings are changed as quickly as possible and only to maintain comfort. Mental health workers, such as a psychiatrist, are available, visiting hours are increased, and religious counselors are given access to the patient. By all reports, such patients generally remain cheerful before lapsing into a coma and dying. Since this article appeared, several other burn units have formally adopted what are called "comfort care protocols." One unit has a detailed, graphic method of deciding the treatment choices for people with burns of varying likelihood of survival. In this hospital, a person who has less than 5 percent chance of survival is offered comfort care alone; but people with 5 to 10 percent chance of survival and whose "specific injuries will drastically affect their quality of life" are also given the choice, as are people who made serious suicide attempts. In a strange twist on the controlling paternalism of medicine, a physician may even prohibit aggressive treatment against a family's or patient's wishes. "This grave risk is rarely taken," the article states, "and then only when compassion clearly demands it."

Comfort care, years later, is still a protocol at only a few burn units. A number of other units practice it, no doubt, in certain select and indisputable cases. Yet few, very few, want to go on record. The publication of that first article, in 1977, was an act of considerable courage on the part of the authors, however sensible and humane their explanation.

As long as the injury is so dreadful that no one is known to have lived through such a thing, these choices are hard to argue against. But many patients who are likely to live also express a wish to die. I am told of a number of patients who, months after their discharge from the hospital, thanked the staff for refusing to let them die when they themselves begged for it. "They know the difference between pain and despair," says one nurse, and I fear she is being a bit glib. Perhaps, lying there, we would all at first want death and then change our minds. Not everyone who survives expresses gratitude. Many spend the rest of their lives trying to find a reason for it. Uncertainty is the birth child of technology, which throws shades of gray in a mechanistic world. This is not unlike the neonatal intensive care unit and its riddles. If not us, who?

Between 1 and 2 percent of the people who suffer severe burns are attempted suicides. This group has a significantly higher death rate during treatment, often because they have made the effort to injure themselves as extensively as possible. Almost all these patients also have a history of previous psychiatric illnesses. Most burn units treat them as aggressively as they would any other patient, assuming that any continued wish to die is, as one article put it, a "manifestation of continued suicidal ideation" and "such a patient should be given compulsory treatment for the psychiatric illness together with essential medical care."

These, too, are good intentions. True, the physician has complete control. True, these patients have lost not just their skin, face, and hands, but their freedom. And true, their intent was subverted by strangers. It is easy for us to say that depression can be treated. We even say it with a touch of impatience. But will we consider what these lucky souls are saved for?

Burn suicides, for two reasons, place themselves in a position of special consideration. The nature of burning, the pain and terror, the primeval destruction wrought— what a masterpiece of symbolic sorrow it is to consign oneself to that fate. To attempt suicide by flames is not simply a matter of escaping despair, but of actually destroying one's self—and doing a near-perfect job of it at that. Most attempted suicides by fire are severely burned. Their cries are not mere "cries for help," minor injuries conveniently discovered before too long. This is kerosene and acid, explosion, cremation. Beyond this must be considered the future. If a young woman swallows a bottle of sleeping pills, she may wake a day or two later without lasting injuries. She will still be without hope, she will still need to claw her way back to life, but she *will* have a body. Burn victims will not. They will have no hands, perhaps, to claw with, no face to face the world with, no voice to cry for help.

On May 21, 1985, Raymond Riles set himself on fire. He sat down in the middle of a pile of papers, books, and bibles and then ignited them; he sat calmly, waiting for death. Riles had waited for death a long time; he is a prisoner on death row in a Texas prison and had grown tired of waiting. The fire was extinguished in time, and Riles was taken to the hospital to recover. Equal access to all, even the damned.

Part of the problem with burn research is the difficulty in following people over a long period of time, but what research has been done appears to indicate that few recovered burn patients kill themselves, even people who had attempted suicide. "We have anecdotal reports of a number of men who struggled with their disfigurement for eight or nine years and then violently killed themselves . . . but these are not proved. . . . More commonly, we hear about people living solitary lives," writes Bernstein. There are no halfway houses for the mutilated— only the great wide world. One must wonder at the fate of the severely burned person who, two years later, has disappeared and is simply considered "lost to follow-up."

In time-honored fashion, stress piles on stress, pain on pain. A man loses his job, then his insurance. The weeks of boredom and discouragement give way to a lethargic hopelessness. He must move to a smaller, older house in a rundown neighborhood, away from his friends. He loses his car. He begins to drink. And the cycle goes round— for months, years, generations. And burns, like almost all accidental injuries, happen with far greater frequency to people under stress in the first place.

House fires, for instance, are more likely to occur in low-income neighborhoods, older houses, and houses with large numbers of people living in them. These houses often have no smoke alarms, and the owners and renters have no insurance. Occupational injuries notwithstanding, almost any kind of burn points a statistical arrow at a group under stress: the poor, the alcoholic and drug addicted, the mentally ill, the unemployed. Often people in these circumstances have more than ordinary difficulty handling the obstacles of adult life. The obstacles presented by a major burn will not be easy to climb.

"Prior to the closure of the burn wound . . . the true personality of the burn patient does not manifest itself," says Jacoby. I was told of a patient who had burned off half his face with a shotgun wound, attempting suicide, who refused plastic surgery on the grounds that he "wanted to look like a Nazi." "A small group has a lot of problems," says a psychologist who works with burn patients. But one study says half have serious psychiatric problems; another says two-thirds. Clearly, not all the problems are "premorbid" (a fine, succinct word), but there appears to be a universal consensus that how well a person coped with stress before the injury is a good predictor of how well he or she will manage the injury itself. A large burn won't necessarily destroy a healthy, well-adjusted person, but a small burn can seriously disrupt a person with other problems.

Lest we forget, it is a "successful adjustment to the sick role" that is the healthiest response. "People just get used to it," a man doing research in adjustment to burns tells me. But another researcher says, "Nothing is known about the psychological outcome of persons who survive major burns."

If there is a best in this world of woe, it is best to be burned very young, to grow up with your scars, and consider them—as much as possible—a part of yourself. It is best to be burned in places like the back, the thighs, parts of our anatomy rarely exposed. It is worst, always, to be burned on the face and the hands or to be burned as a teenager or young adult. For all a child can cry in homesickness, burn pain passes a limit; it violates a child's innocence. Children expect the world to be hard. But this is more than hard. Adults have sinned, if you will. They know about consequences, secrets, and disenchantment. They know, in convoluted ways, without surprise, that pain will come, that there will be suffering. Adults can sense a past without pain and a future without pain, however dimly, in the midst of pain. Children can do none of this; they rise from their beds with the most exhausted and bewildered expressions. Why? And you there, you and you, why do you do this to me? Why won't you stop?

Charlene Kavanaugh, a nurse and burn specialist, developed a new method for dressing changes in children that she believes may relieve some of this terrible wonder. She does this by having the children cause their own pain. Rather than nurturing the child during the procedure (a contradictory behavior at best), she gives the child control and choice: a set schedule, a special "burn care" area, even a "burn care" uniform. The little ones remove their own dressings, wash the wounds, and redress the areas —under supervision and on a time clock. These children, unlike so many others, do not become passive and withdrawn. They will ask questions about disfigurement, discuss the nature of scars. "While there is grief," writes Kavanaugh, "there is not incapacitating withdrawal."

To SURVIVE, ONE MUST FIND THE NAME OF WHAT HAS happened, make attribution, lay blame. Some blame God; others turn to God for solace. Some blame themselves, fate, family, kismet. Nancy blames luck—the bad luck that took her job, took away her insurance, gave her bronchitis, made her take medicine the night her house burned down. Her face is healed over now, although her arms are not, and her face is flushed red and swollen still as the thin scars settle in. With time she will look well enough. The nurse tells me Nancy is depressed, asks for medication in the morning so she can sleep all day. The nurse is impatient with Nancy. "She's thirty going on twelve," she chides.

For others, a bad burn can cleanse, freshen, direct. The flames clear the fallow field for new growth, strike away the weeds that shadow the young tree. This may be what has happened to Luke, who set himself on fire several weeks ago.

He is alert now. His right leg was amputated below the knee, and he lost a toe on the left foot. His stumps will be long in healing because they required grafting, and an artificial leg must wait. "Luke has a positive and constructive attitude toward the future. It's almost as if he is looking forward to the weeks and months ahead. Of course, he barely comprehends what is ahead of him," writes the nurse in charge of Luke's care. "In our observations we see Luke as having experienced a phase where he had 'nothing to live for'—no goals and objectives set for himself. Now that he has survived his injury he has goals and tasks he wants to achieve. His new physical state has forced goals upon him which he has accepted. Now we see a very motivated young man."

"I am sending a thank you to all of you in the Burn Unit for the special care and love you gave." "How could we possibly express our feelings and gratitude to all of you sufficiently?" "Not a night goes by that I don't think of all of you hard at work." "Thanks for taking good care of my baby." These are excerpts from letters written by former patients and their families to the staff of one burn unit.

Little Michael went home with his father today, just a month after the fire. His is an unusual recovery, rapid and uncomplicated. It's far from over, of course: he will wear pressure garments on his chest and hands for another eighteen months, and stockings or a mask on his face.

Zero mistakes. Jered is still alive. His burn wounds are almost healed, but he remains in critical condition and he is still on the ventilator. "His lungs are like those of a sixty-year-old man with chronic lung disease," says the head nurse. The smoke inhalation, the high oxygen, the ventilator pressures have all caused permanent damage. To wean him off the machine will require "accepting lower oxygen levels" in his blood than one wants a child to have. We are in the neonatal unit once again, and no one wants to stop. Jered has been saved from certain death only to be consigned to an uncertain life, to be a respirator baby. His bill is past six figures, and who will pay? For that matter, what are we afraid of? He opens his eyes when you call his name; he winces with pain. These are the positive signs. No one has investigated the damage to his brain; no EEG yet. I wonder why. Would it only add another shade of gray?

O N CHRISTMAS EVE JERED'S UNIT ADMITTED ANOTHER pair of siblings, also victims of a house fire, also severely burned and on ventilators. "You walked on your tiptoes through the module, it was so hard," the nurse says. "We had a difficult holiday."

Sherry has gone home; she's started school again. She wears her pressure stockings, a net cap on her head. Come this summer she'll have a toe-to-hand transplant to gain back a thumb that never healed. She holds her head high, walking between classes. I imagine the litany she sings under her breath: "Less rigid, less red, less dry." I hope she remembers the caresses that accompanied it. Her trial isn't over.

How *can* we comprehend what lies ahead? Children can be so cruel; adults in their cowardice can be even more so. Bernstein tells a little story in passing: "James was a fourteen-year-old who had sustained facial and neck burns in a house fire. He returned to school, where he had always been a marginal student. When he was called on in class and failed to answer a question, the teacher asked, 'What's the matter? Did they also burn your brains out?' "

T HE WORLD HAS ALWAYS HAD THE OCCASIONAL FREAK, the Elephant Man and rubber-faced woman, the extraordinarily tall and immensely fat, and these people have held some kind of oddly privileged status in history. Appearing singly, without explanation, they pique our pity and curiosity without any true threat. They are the modern Minotaur, symbols of good and evil, reduced to mortal status and stripped of his mystic powers. Like Janelle's more rudely made cousins, freaks satisfy our anthropomorphism, help us draw the circle tighter, define the boundaries. We haven't learned tolerance from mutation, only a kind of self-centered gratitude.

Such can never be the case for the burned, because they are our own creation. I have to think, tritely, of the banishments and persecution that lepers suffered because they had a deformity that could be caught, a contamination. Like leprosy, burns are a contamination, a contagion—an extremity that could strike us all. We turn away from a man in his thirties, both legs missing, as he wheels down the street because, however unconsciously, we fear he is a war veteran—a product. No simple genetic mystery here. So we turn from the burned with a quiver of the stomach, fearing for ourselves—our own special creation.

Burned people only want their lives back. They want to live next door to us, shop at our stores, attend our schools, marry us. Are we asking too much of them, to make them try? Are we asking too much of ourselves? The subconscious terror fades so slowly. We gladly, gleefully, invite them to return from the dead (no, we insist), and then, holding the power of excommunication in the palms of our hands, we send them out alone. Perhaps those who not only survive in some contentment but thrive after a major burn are pilgrims in the wilderness, seeking the deeper meanings. Perhaps they are hallowed in some way by the shock of those around them, as though by a rarefied, ice-cold wind that etches away the rough edges.

It is a new world they have passed into: "I am fire and air; my other elements I give to baser life."

THE GORDIAN KNOT

CREAKING AND SLIDING, OUR BODIES EDGE TOWARD OB-livion. So many forces come to bear: gravity, with its steady, silent pull; friction and the heat it generates; sorrow and desire and time, bruising us and making demands. The little, lithe inventions we hide under our skin are slowly worked from volcanic angles into Appalachian mounds, soft and worthless. Time is the surgeon's reason, the surgeon's point—to shore up the cliffs that inevitably erode away.

In the hierarchy of medicine, the surgeon ranks high. In the hierarchy of surgery, he is king. Everyone else is below. Let me generalize a bit about the surgeon, who is almost always a man. He is brusque, hurried, subject to fits of pique and a short temper, suspicious of new faces and questions. He is a man with a mission and doors to go through. These doors swing only one way—inward—and close behind him even if someone else is following.

Surgeons are accustomed to being waited on—it is the point of their work—and this expectation continues outside the operating room. They see patients as problems to be solved and other health professionals as their auxiliary staff. Much of the doctor-as-confessor, doctor-as-poet literature has been written by surgeons, who feel a bit defensive and seek to justify themselves, explain their craft as art. Surgeons like shine and steel and clear equations; they make neat slices and fine cuts and are not given to ambivalence or vacillation—at least, not given to show it. They reinvent the body in their own image.

Unlike medicine, surgery is by necessity a mechanistic discipline. Medicine chooses, tries, to be mechanistic, but the opaqueness of the body and the stubborn subjective notions of patients can frustrate that. "Life is biochemistry," a medical student tells me, but he knows it's not that easy. Surgery has an undeniable certainty that medicine lacks; it seeks to simplify the general by illuminating the specific. Life may be partly biochemical, but in the operating room it is carpentry, plumbing, and sculpture, a physical vocation, a putting to right of that which is disordered. The hierarchy has a purpose, and it is not only to make clear the duties of each person in the room for efficiency's sake. It serves to structure the work itself, to provide the delineation such work requires.

In every "operating suite," as the series of rooms and tiled hallways and dressing areas are called, there is a lounge for the nurses and a lounge for the doctors. The nurses' rooms have lockers and shelves, rows and rows of tennis shoes and boots and white shoes, pieces of uniform and sweaters and jackets hung on hooks, piles of green and blue scrubs (yellow and pink if you're lucky) on shelves, boxes of shoe covers, hats to hold your hair in, and masks. There is a bathroom, a pot of coffee, a few stale doughnuts, perhaps a microwave oven, yesterday's newspaper, several ashtrays, and a bulletin board.

I don't know what doctors' lounges look like; I've never seen one, never cared to look.

Somewhere in the maze of halls whose walls and floors shine as only walls and floors washed every day can shine is one or more rows of sinks. The sinks are broad and deep, looked over by big steel faucets. You turn the water on and off with your knee, squirt out soap using a button under your foot. Everyone washes here, but the doctors wash together. They talk about the surgery that just ended, the next one to come. Always I see men at the sinks, the hair on their arms wet and dripping.

This is my generalization, my distance. Surgeons often seem very different from me—in a fundamental way—in how they see the world. I know all generalities fail eventually; individuals intrude and break the rules. Surgeons are no more or less frail than the rest of us, no more or less wise. One way or the other, we all try to put to rights that which we find disordered.

THERE'S A PROBLEM WITH THE LAB RESULTS. MARTHA Carroll, a seventy-nine-year-old woman with arthritis in both hips, lies on the small high table in the center of the total hip operating room, waiting. Surgery is scheduled to begin at 8:00 A.M., in fifteen minutes, but a vital point of order, her potassium blood level, is missing from the chart. Skip, the circulating nurse, makes several phone calls. The results are finally found—below normal. Skip looks at Les, the scrub nurse who is steadily opening packages for his long table of tools. No surgery if the potassium is too low; it risks heart problems.

The anesthesiologist bangs out of the room, angry. No excuse for this clerical error. The deficiency should have been spotted and corrected last night. Les keeps opening packages, laying out rows of instruments, lethal-looking knives, sabers, drills, and saws, basins and sponges and packages of needles and thread, a mortar and pestle, a line of pliers. Skip stands beside the sleeping Martha, holding her hand. She has arthritis in both hips; the position she holds can't be comfortable.

(I asked a nurse who worked in a recovery room, guarding over people fresh from surgery and still dim, why she didn't prefer the actual operating room. "Surgery nursing," she replied with a slight and delicate sneer, "is high-tech Stepin Fetchit.")

I stand, scrubbed, gowned, and masked, by the door. Beside me is a very tall young fellow named Mark, a physical therapy student who has never seen surgery before and has been sent by his professors for initiation. Everyone is here—Martha, Skip, Les, Mark, and me—everyone but the surgeon and the anesthesiologist.

More phone calls. Where's Dr. Acheson, the surgeon? He hates to start late. Word comes that the anesthesiologist refuses to work the operation; Acheson wants to go ahead. After forty-five minutes of negotiation, another anesthesiologist strides into the room. She is thin and pretty and dark-skinned, black curls straying from under her cap. Les calls out a greeting; she deflects it sharply. "I'm angry, so don't talk to me." She takes her seat at the head of the table and begins to sort through the vials of medication. At 9:10, Dr. Acheson arrives, trailing a resident behind him.

Dr. Carl Acheson is known as Dr. A to the people who work with him regularly. He is a man of medium height, in his late forties, cheerful and rushed. "Let's get started," he calls to everyone in the room, feeling that lost hour of argument behind him. "Skip, call my office and cancel the ankle we were going to do this afternoon. It's too late now."

He moves to the light screen at one end of the room,

pushing his glasses back up to his nose, where they rest against the edge of his mask. In this room, compulsively clean, ordinary surgical masks are not enough. The costumes render the point of gender almost moot. Over the cap goes a hat that covers the mouth, nose, and neck like a ski mask, so that only the eyes are visible. Dr. A takes the silhouette of Mrs. Carroll's right hip and compares it to a chart of artificial hips, making pencil scratches along the edge of a transparent ruler. He chooses a size and calls the code number to Les, who picks yet another package out of a pile and lays it on the table. The two surgeons leave to scrub while Martha is finally put to sleep.

SURGERY IS MARKED BY THE STANDARDS OF SOMETHING called "sterile technique": a set of rules by which people and things and sometimes entire rooms are demarcated "clean" and "sterile." No, it doesn't always make sense that one's chest is sterile but one's side is dirty, that the table is sterile only to its edge, or that pouring liquids from a height necessarily keeps them from becoming contaminated. But most of these rules hold true most of the time; the point is standardization. A surgeon can travel the world over and find other surgeons and nurses who will do the same thing the same way. It helps line up the borders squarely—that it is always done this way. Only inside the wound, a wound he has made, must the surgeon face real uncertainty.

Almost every operation has at least one scrub nurse, who washes and gowns sterile like the surgeon and is responsible for setting up the tables of instruments, preparing sterile materials, handing tools to the physician—often anticipating the next request silently. Likewise, operations are attended by a circulating nurse, who is clean but not sterile. She is responsible for getting equipment, preparing the patient, opening packages, answering the phone, emptying wastebaskets, and myriad other tasks. The scrub nurse and circulating nurse together count sponges and needles before and after surgery to be certain everything that goes into the patient also comes out. At the head of the table sits the anesthesiologist, responsible for monitoring the patient's life signs and level of consciousness and for keeping careful records of the drugs and blood given. Complex surgeries often have one or more surgical assistants (often residents in training) and extra nurses. Simple surgeries may use a nurse-anesthetist, specially trained but less expensive than the physician-anesthesiologist. Like many surgeons, Acheson tries to work with the same nurses as often as possible. He is a hip man and only a hip man, and there's nothing simple about hip surgery, simple as it may appear. Every bit of extra experience will eventually come in handy.

The hip, at its best, is a free ball and socket, a slide-and-glide joint, with a nearly spherical femoral head (the top of the thigh bone) riding in a matching bowl of bone called the acetabulum. Both start out smooth and opalescent, a happy pair. Time, friction, and gravity work their refinements on all of us. For some, the inflammation of arthritis creates a new cycle of bone growth and calluses, irritation and pain. Always pain. Arthritis is incurable and progressive (in the system of medical thought), and in the elderly it can mean the end of an active life. Drugs ease pain but can't repair the damage. Thus the surgeon's solution to the problem of the Gordian knot: instead of trying to unravel the puzzle, simply cut it away.

M ARTHA GOES SILENTLY TO SLEEP AS THE HYPNOTIC drug slides into her vein. Quickly she is draped in sterile blue, all but a leg and belly, a curtain propped up above her neck so the anesthesiologist can watch her face while the operation proceeds. Skip inserts a catheter to drain off her urine and scrubs her right leg—from waist to toe—with a foaming antiseptic, brown like grasshopper juice. He scrubs from the center out, top down, many times. Her leg is hung in a sling while he works, around and around. When Skip has finished the scrub, he wraps her foot and lower leg in another blue drape.

Dr. A backs into the OR, hands dripping, and Les hands him a sterile towel, a gown to fold into, and a pair of gloves, one at a time. He is followed by the anonymous surgical resident who will assist. They take their places, one on each side.

Martha is humped up on her side, the right leg now pulled far over the left in an awkward, unbalanced tangle. She is only a leg now and that blue, in the field of blue, the blue gowns and masks, the blue-draped tables covered with tools. Mark is placed, like a swordbearer in a Shakespearean tableau, beside the resident. I stand like a lady-in-waiting beside Acheson. We form a full circle of germlessness, blue, crinkly, careful. He takes the scalpel and cuts—the top of the hip to a third of the way down the thigh—and cuts again through the globular yellow fat, and deeper. The resident follows with a cautery, holding tiny spraying blood vessels and burning them shut with an electric current. One small, throbbing arteriole escapes, and his glasses and cheek are splattered.

When the skin and fat are pulled away, the tendons can be seen, tight and drawn, and the thin, long muscles that pull the leg outward, backward, and forward. Acheson cuts the small outermost ones and then begins to pull the others aside, one by one. A bit of pelvic bone can be seen at the top of the incision; into this Acheson hammers a long steel pin, rap, rap, and the table shakes. "A landmark," he says, "to make sure I don't lengthen or shorten her leg too much."

"I DIDN'T WANT TO TAKE CARE OF CANCER, AND I DIDN'T want to take care of dying people," Acheson now says about his choice, many years ago, of orthopedics. "In orthopedics you get to work with kids, young adults. And I do carpentry, too, so I like the hands-on work." The similarities are undeniable. His name comes up quickly in conversations about surgeons; he is respected as well as popular. The nurses kid him more than many other doctors. They kid, but there's no back talk. Acheson carries an authority into the operating theater. Things are done his way, but if a surprise rears up or a mistake is made, he'll say his piece and drop the subject. He likes to talk while he works; money problems interest him. Like almost every physician I've ever met, if he's interested in the subject, he'll dominate the conversation.

Acheson says money is the only problem with hips anymore. The technology has improved a great deal in the eleven years total hip implants have been done in the United States, but the costs remain untenably high. The surgery itself is complex, and the follow-up is long, requiring special nursing care and rehabilitation to be certain of success. But Medicare reimburses both physician and hospital only $2165.90 per hip in Acheson's city, a loss of several thousand dollars when compared to privately paying patients. The implant itself, that piece of metal, costs another $1800. Often, Acheson adds, he must release a patient after doing one hip and readmit him or her later for the other, because otherwise the physician would be paid for only one. Surgeons in the United States perform between 80,000 and 90,000 total hip implants every year, at a cost in the billions.

"Why do we have to cut costs?" he asks the room while he cuts a hip. "Why don't we quit building bombers and spend the money to help people have a better quality of life?" It is a hypothetical question, but he incites response. His resident, with an edge of wariness, begins an argument about tort law and liability. Acheson likes to talk about lawsuits too, and soon the conversation is crowded, full of interruptions and an occasional comment on the progress of the operation.

Dr. A anticipates an interesting case tomorrow, when he will try to repair another surgeon's mistakes. A young woman, he begins, had polio as a child. She walked with a light limp and a click in one hip when she squatted. That was all. During a company physical, though, a physician told her that without hip implants she would be bedridden within a year. She had both hips replaced, a few weeks later, by a physician without much experience in the area, and then she *was* bedridden and in pain. She sued and won ("Not enough," says Acheson), and tomorrow he will try to repair the damage, return some function, and lessen her pain.

Acheson has two basic criteria to determine if patients need a hip replaced. First, they have to ask for it, showing him that the situation bothers them enough to seek help. Second, they need to be well enough to come into his office for a consultation, showing him they have enough vigor to be surgical candidates. If everything else bears out, Acheson considers it a medically necessary operation. But he admits that until recently he shied away from the very elderly.

"I had a case—would you say a woman in her nineties should have a total hip? Is it worthwhile?" Another hypothetical question. He describes an operation he performed on a senile woman of ninety-three. The family, who cared for the woman at home, and their family physician had to coax Acheson for months before he consented to the risky surgery. He was surprised and pleased to receive a long thank-you letter from her family a few months later, explaining that with the decrease in pain and improved mobility, the woman's mood had improved and she was much easier to care for. She would be able to continue living at home instead of moving to a nursing home as had been feared.

A FTER ABOUT THIRTY MINUTES, THE HIP JOINT IS FREED from its tight cover of muscle. It lies quiescent. Then the surgeons pick up the leg and together give it a forcible twist, putting their backs into it, until the bone dislocates with a slurpy pop and the thighbone snaps free of its acetabular nest. The leg is propped on a nearby table at an odd angle, the foot twisted, the round femoral head at the end of the bone peering out at the world. It is like an accident scene, this bloody limb below a bloody hole, with four hands buried in it.

Mark, who is very tall, seems suddenly to sway where he stands. Skip, whose eyes move around the room without rest, searching for the next chore, has seen all this before. He knows how people who have never seen a surgery before can react to this particular one. He is at Mark's side, gently guiding him away.

"I'm just going to sit down here for a while," Mark tells everyone, unnecessarily. He slumps in the chair by the door, his forehead pale, and then he leans forward, head between his knees. Acheson cuts, and no one comments for a minute; then, one by one, each person in the room tells a little story, self-effacing, about his or her first witnessing of an operation, the nausea, the disbelief. It is a bow to Mark and his embarrassment; surgeons, medical students, and nurses get faint too.

I actually did faint once, years ago. I remember going down so very carefully, conscious as I fell that all about me were tables draped with sterile tools, that I mustn't touch them, mustn't grab. I thoughtfully folded my legs underneath me, curling up on the cool and soothing floor—I'd gotten so warm, suddenly, like a Victorian maiden. The humiliation was acute, especially because the surgery hadn't yet begun. I'd been watching, for the first time, the administration of a spinal anesthetic. The patient, nine months pregnant and about to have a cesarean, hunched over on herself on the side of the table while the anesthesiologist searched for a certain space between her vertebrae. She slid in the long, long needle and then withdrew it. That wasn't the space. And she did it again, and again, and each time as she pulled out the needle a round drop of dark red blood pooled where the needle had been. Each time, as five minutes, then ten minutes went by, the heavy, cumbersome woman moaned. Finally she began saying, "Don't, please don't," each time the needle dove into her spine. That's when I fainted. I haven't again, nor have I forgotten; I feel nothing but sympathy for Mark.

WITH A THIN-BLADED ELECTRIC SAW, THE SURGEONS slice off the top of the femur, and Dr. A hands the uneven globe to Les, who will later give it to the organ bank technicians for use in a bone graft. The ball is rough and shows feeble attempts at repairs, little sharp abutments of bone that only increased Martha's pain. Taking a ridged metal bore and hooking it to a drill, Dr. A reams the femoral canal, forcing the marrow out of the center of the bone with a whirring of metal and the sound of construction. "We're delicate surgeons here," he laughs as he leans into the work, the wound filling with blood and marrow. Then he turns to the acetabulum, chipping the biggest irregularities out with a hammer and edge, finally sanding it back to a soft pearly surface. The blood and bits of bone and marrow are washed away with a jet of water, the spray sucked back into a vacuum tube. Occasionally an acetabulum itself is so damaged it must be created, a difficult job. "The people who are hurt bad enough to have a broken acetabulum used to die. But now our trauma teams can save them, so we're faced with some very tricky surgeries." The room is hot, and after a complaint, Acheson takes his gloved hand out of the wound long enough to demonstrate convection currents to all who listen. The heat rests just above the wound, in our faces, filled with the wet, rich smell of blood and muscle. He has a long, bloody glob of fat stuck to his shoe, and as he shifts his feet, the fat wiggles. Talk and jokes continue, a discussion of the hospital's new administration mingling with an argument over the relative salaries of nurses and physicians.

The canal is clean and well-worked, the bowl of bone satiny smooth. Les prepares the glue as Dr. A fiddles with the new acetabulum. It is an admirable piece of work, a shiny patellar steel, a white socket with a roughened gray metallic backing. Several small plastic plugs jut out of the metal to form a structure for the grout to ride in, so that time and friction won't wear it all away. He sets it in and peers at it; then he pulls it out again.

Les mixes the glue by pouring together a liquid and powder that combine in an exothermic reaction, releasing energy in the form of heat. Rapidly the glue becomes first a syrup, then a paste, and then a thick cement, and Les counts the time: "Four minutes. Nine minutes." At a precise thickness, he hands the mixture to the surgeon and

Acheson slathers it in the bowl. Without pausing, he slaps the artificial cup on top of bone and the grout squirts out from beneath it.

"Not too much, get the extra there," he instructs the resident. This is similar to the glue used by dentists for crowns, and it has a sickening chemical odor. Ten minutes after the mixture was made, the excess is a rock-hard white mass, still so hot it can barely be held.

Using a dummy prosthesis, the surgeons fit a new femur into the prepared canal and pop the leg together again. Acheson measures—the leg is 2 centimeters longer now, too long. He pulls out the dummy, and they saw away more of the thigh bone, working it down to an edge. Again, a third time, the leg is put together, taken apart, as if by children trying to figure out how it worked. When the leg is within a centimeter of its original length, it is time for the true implant. Again the glue is mixed—each surgery uses about $120 worth of glue—and the artificial hip is produced, sterile and fresh. It is a shining femur, newly born, with a perfectly round and silky steel head, and more of the roughened silver plate on the long bone, to hold the cement in its tiny grooves.

The mechanical man, jerry-built. While the artificial heart raises hackles and the search for an artificial kidney just muddies the water, tens of thousands of people walk around on artificial hips; thousands more lift and throw with artificial elbows. Why does one disturb and the other comfort? Is it just the price, the theatrics, the overblown derring-do of the heart surgeons on the newscasts? Do I simply dislike the flamboyant defiance of certain death? Or is it the purpose? I wonder if some of Acheson's contentment with his work comes from the unequivocal nature of his particular cunning and what it buys for people. No one's hanging around afterward to ask difficult questions about hip surgeries; their worth is unquestioned.

The canal is first packed with a plug of cement to keep

the implant from working its way down. Acheson places the stake in its channel, and for the last time, the dislocated limb is returned to order. The surgeons play with its range of motion, moving the leg here, there, in directions it hasn't moved for years. Then the sharp wound is slowly stitched. Duration—almost three hours from the first slice.

"She'll be in less pain tomorrow than she was this morning," Acheson predicts. "We don't worry about pneumonia in our patients because they're up and walking as soon as we let them."

He complains a bit more about money as he stitches. Each medical instrument company that manufactures tools for hip surgeries makes a complete set, and they don't fit each other; the doctor must buy an entire set from one manufacturer. Much of the equipment is disposable and must be replaced for every operation. Acheson says that for years, he used an inexpensive saw bought from a department store. Finally, the hospital told him to buy a standard medical model, which cost over $4000. The water spray that cleans the wound could be replaced by a Water Pic, he adds—but Water Pic hasn't got Underwriters Laboratories approval. The costs of that testing come high. He shakes his head and sews.

On the wall of the room under the telephone is taped a headline cut from an alternative newspaper. Its edges are frayed, the paper a little yellowed. It reads "Hip Capitalism."

NEEDLES IN THE FACE

I HOLD THE POLARITY CLOSE TO HEART, I ADMIT, THIS distance between myself and surgeons—and all physicians. I expect to be disrespected, so when I'm close to surgeons I am ready for irreconcilable differences. There is a bit of pleasure, warped though it may be, in sparring. But I can spar only as a visitor, a guest—like the recovery room nurse, I would never fit in as an assistant. I am almost ready, though, to admit the exceptions.

Dr. Acheson is one, and Bob Nieland is another. Nieland fixes eyes, and he's a man who loves his work. Like Acheson he is blessed with a skill remarkably lacking in controversy. The arguments are technical, practical, this tool or that timing. No major ethical dramas here. Today Bob Nieland has offered to show me the secret of his gleeful manner, the reason for his pleasure. He's going to show me eyes.

Forced to lose one of our senses, few of us would choose to lose our sight. Rather farewell to the sound of symphonies, the stroke of skin, the taste of chocolate, or smell of fresh-baked bread than to lose our sight. Everything about us lives in that realm; we find our place in the world in relation to what we see around us. We describe mysteries with metaphors of blindness: the hidden, the shadowed, the hooded, the veiled, the eclipsed. Newly blind people adjust to a world that is shaped differently, adjust to their own new shape. We lose vision and gain radar, but it's a trade only a few would make.

The human eye is a structure daring in its simplicity, a mere oval globe with a lens hanging over a pool of sticky fluid that focuses rays on a thousand tiny cells. The eye is an original mirror, moved hither and yon by little muscles that push and pull it to face the desired. We filter the world into a prism that fractures and splinters color without sensation, without consciousness, at the speed of light.

The lens of the human eye is less than half an inch in diameter. Clear as glass, it sits behind the accordian iris that stretches and shrinks like elastic to control the light. The iris is the color of the eye, and the lens behind it is dark with the retina and sight. The lens is two-thirds water and one-third protein, and it is joined to the surface of the eyeball by the suspensory ligaments, which allow it to hang lightly, relaxed. Encased in a soft capsule womb, the lens has no pain fibers, no blood vessels. It is nourished by the placental aqueous humor, watery and thin, in the anterior chamber in front and by the vitreous humor, thick and viscous, in the posterior chamber behind. When the muscles of the eye contract and relax the suspensory ligaments, the lens bulges and flattens in order to focus on the object at hand. It is a tool, a pawn, to catch and move the image until it clicks into sharpness against the retina and is recognized.

Until we hit middle age, that is. Then a certain amount of stiffness and clouding of the lens settles in—"senile cataract." Unflattering by name, but nothing to interfere with vision. We get bifocals and go about our business. That may be the worst our eyes will offer us, and it may not. True cataracts drop a film of jelly across the lens, clouding out vision altogether, painlessly, insidiously, maddeningly unstoppable. Babies are sometimes born with cataracts, and they can grow from poison, electric shock, diabetes, infections, and trauma. In 1970, cataracts were the second leading cause of blindness in the United States—but in 1982, 600,000 cataracts were surgically removed. This is the most common major surgery paid for by Medicare. Here is a miracle of the twentieth century: a person essentially blind for years may see again after half an hour in routine surgery.

B OB NIELAND PERFORMS ABOUT 300 CATARACT SURGER-ies a year. Surgery and teaching others his technique for inserting artificial lenses are all he does. Nieland is in the vanguard of posterior intraocular lens implants—IOLs—a surgery still under investigation by the Food and Drug Administration despite the fact that 69 percent of the lens implants in the United States are now of this type. IOLs have changed the face of cataract operations.

Nieland is a small, bouncy man in late middle age, slightly graying and neat in his movements, with glasses over his bright eyes. He moves quickly, talking to himself when not in conversation with others. Nieland has a good working relationship with a small private hospital happy to have his steady business; there he has his own operating theater, with two regular nurses and a bank of videotaping equipment hooked to his refrigerator-sized microscope. It is a place he feels at home.

Who wants a knife in the eye? I would choose to sleep through this procedure, dreaming about Dr. Sassall and where he lives. But cataract patients are usually elderly —86 percent are over sixty-five years of age—and are not a group popular with anesthesiologists. The elderly face considerable risks from anesthesia, which can slow the breathing and make the heart beat irregularly. Over the years, a new form of anesthesia has developed, resulting in a cocktail of tranquilizers and relaxants that send the patient into a quiet fog of amnesia through which they can answer and cooperate without awareness. The amnesia, an anesthesiologist assures me, is certain: patients really don't remember the pain or the surgery. Can there be pain without the memory of it? Does it matter? Can it still hurt us? Still I squirm.

Today's first patient, one of five, is rolled into the operating room already drowsy and dressed for surgery with his hair bundled under a blue cap. He slowly, languidly, answers to his name in a bass voice. He is seventy-three years old and couldn't care less right now. The nurses slide him onto the table in the bright white room while Nieland fits a tape into the video machine and then hurriedly seats himself at the head of the table. He will lean over the patient's face, upside-down, for the whole procedure.

Nieland takes a large syringe and needle and sticks it into the man's face between his cheek and ear, beside his brow. The man winces slightly and then is still while the doctor injects a local anesthetic and then unscrews the syringe, leaving the needle sticking out into space from the man's skin. He screws on another syringe and injects more; then he pulls the mess out and waits a moment— just a moment. Without further prelude, Nieland pulls back the upper eyelid of the man lying below him and inserts a needle behind the eyeball. The man lies motionless, staring. He moves the needle here and there, injecting the various sections of musculature, and then he unceremoniously closes the eye and rubs it with a mercury weight, forcing the drug into the tissue and softening the eye for its coming trial. He must lower the pressure that keeps the eye firm or else the structure would pop its segments out during the operation. The circulating nurse takes his place with the weight, and he leaves without a backward glance, trotting out to scrub up.

Until very recently, most cataracts were removed, and that was that; the eye was left without a lens. For focus the patient had to rely on a pair of exceedingly thick "cataract glasses," through which only the object directly in front could be seen, as at the end of a tunnel of clarity. Peripheral vision was lost, and in effect, a filmy blindness was traded for a circular window, a periscope picture. Contact lenses seemed to hold promise, but they were a failure with an older population poorly suited to the fine muscle movements and motor control needed to care for and insert contacts. Before even this much vision was returned, the person was forced to retreat into complete blindness as the cataract "ripened," becoming fully mature and opaque, easier to remove in its hardness.

Finer instruments make it possible now to break the capsule and remove the lens before it is fully stiff, so cataracts can be removed as soon as they begin to interfere with normal life. And now lenses are put *in* the eye permanently, making glasses and contacts obsolete. The artificial lens is stiff but clear, transparent but still unable to focus. Nieland and his patients talk before surgery about the person's particular needs—are they readers, gardeners? Must they drive? Nieland chooses a primary focus, short or long, and orders a lens of that curvature. Secondary focus is provided by ordinary bifocal glasses.

Complications of varying degrees are fairly common, but failures are few after thirty years of research, most of it on the eyes of rabbits.

With Nieland and Susan, the scrub nurse, clean and hunched up to the table, surgery begins. A translucent plastic shroud is draped over the patient's entire body, supported by a rigid bar above his chin that breathes oxygen into the womb it creates. You can vaguely see his moist shape, still and solemn, in its tent. Only an oval cutout over the left eye is open. The room lights are dimmed to darkness and the ponderous electric microscope is rolled into place over the hole. A single, sharp beam of light comes to rest on that eye. Nieland has one foot on a button under the table to turn the videotape machine on and off. The circulating nurse will fiddle with the pause and focus. "I have a lecture tomorrow and I need some pictures," he says to everyone, and the screen clicks into life. At the foot of the bed an eye 2 feet across and 1 foot high springs forth, staring at the shape of its owner.

Nieland pulls back the lids and squints into the pupil, humming, and then he reaches for the tiny retractors Susan is already holding toward him. He draws the lids back with the forked instruments and secures them, revealing a white sphere that is too big, like that of poor Robert, his eyelid burned away. Drops of salt solution pour steadily over its surface, keeping it moist, its delicate cells alive. Later this solution will run inside the eye itself, replacing the humor that drains from the cuts. Nieland has done this a thousand times and more; there is no hesitation as he leans against the eye with a scalpel, watching his hands through the microscope.

"This is the safest surgery in the world," he says happily. He claims for his own practice a complication rate of less than 1 percent—far below average. The FDA's continuing investigation irks him considerably.

In a few moments Nieland has cut under the cornea, the outer surface of the eye, and into the anterior chamber. He nicks the iris a bit, and a smear of brown slides across the white. The largest portion of time is spent in carefully releasing the lens and the front half of the capsule from its position while avoiding any tear in the back wall behind. The process is called "expression." "It takes a certain touch," says Nieland.

In ten minutes the lens is free, and it pops suddenly out and up above the surface. It is a hard yellow little pill, slippery and rough. I rescue it from its fate in the wastebasket and squeeze it between my fingertips, where its crushes softly into a waxy film.

The small slice in the eye is closed with a quick stitch, and with a tool very like a large needle Nieland slides inside the chamber and vacuums out the torn portions of capsule. The steel tube slips in and out, and the patches of tissue ride up an almost-perfect vacuum. Nieland helped create this particular tool. A quick buzz now and then signals the whir and click of a camera mounted on the microscope, and the picture on the video screen starts, stops, and reverses, Dali-like, the eye whole, then in pieces, then whole again.

"In India they don't use anesthesia," says Nieland, chatty during this routine chore. "People just walk in and lie down in the middle of the day. And they hold perfectly still." I can't tell if he admires that discipline or pities the passivity.

The inside of the cornea is a layer of cells extremely sensitive to touch. Normally the cornea is held aloft by the aqueous humor, underwater, and thus protected. If the artificial lens, made of a plastic called polymethyl methacrylate, were to scrape that inner surface, it could permanently damage the cornea and cause a different kind of blindness, one much harder to cure. Even in the most successful implants, the cornea often develops a "foreign-body reaction" in response to the lens.

To cushion the cells, then, Nieland injects a bubble of air into the chamber that rises against the transparent cornea. The larger-than-life eye on the video screen looks out at us, brightly lit, with an air bubble inside, trapped under the quick-frozen ice. Nieland watches his hands, hardly pausing, embroidering swiftly like the seamstress who gossips as she works. "Gosh," he says with a smile, "I like my work."

The artificial lens itself is a shiny clear circle, slightly curved, with two filaments that wind out from opposing sides like the spiral arms of a pinwheel. The filaments anchor the lens behind the iris, where it is held between the far wall of the capsule and the iris. The lens costs about $300 now, although Nieland anticipates the price will drop to about $100 very soon. He has invented a tool called the Shooter to "inject" the lens behind the iris. It slides through the cornea, under the pillow of air, and the iris stretches at an odd sharp angle to accommodate its entrance and then snaps back into place as Nieland releases the lens.

N IELAND IS PAID ABOUT $1800 FOR THE SURGERY, WHICH includes the six months of postoperative care and care for any complications. A report issued in July, 1985, by a Congressional subcommittee states that almost half of the $3.5 billion Medicare spends on cataract surgeries every year is wasted through kickbacks and fraud. The report accuses manufacturers of offering physicians a variety of rewards—resort condominiums, the use of yachts—for buying a particular product. Nieland performs a surgery that is rarely in headlines, without the slightly skewed discomfort of heroics. Unfortunate that its mundane character is marred by greed. Nieland himself says he is overpaid for his work.

Nieland slips the needle under the cornea one more time, shattering the air pocket like glass before withdrawing the tiny pieces; as he pulls out the air, the solution is fed in, filling up the pool again. He stitches the cornea shut, over and under in an awkward, uneven cross-stitch. There is a fringe benefit to this surgery: it corrects many cases of nearsightedness and farsightedness—and by the tension in the stitches he is making now, Nieland can correct much astigmatism, the curious distorted focus due to an irregularly shaped eyeball. He will see the patient in his office many times in the next few months. If astigmatism is still a problem, Nieland can sit the man down and loosen or tighten a few stitches then and there to try to correct the problem. Snipping a single stitch may be all that is needed. "I get them down as close to zero as possible," says Nieland, "because it's fun."

Sewing done, the single exposed eye is thickly patched, the anesthesiologist withdraws his drugs, and the patient stirs. He is wheeled, groggy, to the recovery room down the hall, and if all goes well, he will return home this afternoon. He will have a swollen, droopy, mucky eye for a while, as if an inflamed fist hit him. For a month he will wear glasses at all times during the day and a shield at night to keep him protected from a bump or unconscious scratching. After five weeks, the eye is normal—normal! And he can drive, dance, cook, make love. It is, as Alfred Lord Tennyson says, "a sight to make an old man young."

Nieland and Acheson are making routine what was impossible a short while ago. They are amiable men in a rude profession. Again I remember Sassall, who lives "just under and behind" his eyes. How would he submit to Nieland's needle? Could any restored skill be worth the rape? Or does any chance at sight make any violation worthwhile to a man who lives in his eyes? I wonder at those who live inside their beating hearts; I wonder at this regulating of the extraordinary. If I live in my heart, what does an artificial one offer me? Nothing, nothing at all, no womb. Where, rising from that sickbed, could I live?

THE MAN WHO WASN'T THERE

S TATISTICS ARE THE MEAT OF MEDICINE, WHETHER THEY define pain and all its prosaic descriptions or enumerate one's chances of getting out alive. The patient and his or her relevant pieces are assimilated into the data of survival rates and side-effect frequency. Like weather predictions, every step is stamped with percentages; each treatment is laden with possibility, pregnant with cost-benefit ratios. Freak accidents and miracles are everyday stuff in the computer. Spend a long enough time in your sickbed and you'll be visited by one or the other; spend a long enough time and you become a case history just for being there on rounds the next day—and the next.

A NN BURKE IS A PRACTICAL WOMAN, FAST-TALKING AND quick to get to the point of a conversation. She is no-nonsense in the flesh, wanting even the jokes she tells to be over and done with as efficiently as possible. Ann is the head nurse of a busy cancer ward, stout and ruddy with her direct, impatient face framed by short, dark hair. She does the many small tasks of her job in a linear fashion, without pause. Monday is always her worst day, with papers piled up and often several new patients who arrived over the weekend.

In the first room is a teenage boy dying of leukemia. His curtains are drawn, and he speaks in the slow, rounded tones of the drugged, complaining of pain. Ann tells him she'll be back. Next door is Carl Burger, a fifty-nine-year-old man whose colon cancer has metastasized to his lungs and brain, grown vine-like and tenacious. He has been unable to drink or eat enough at home, and his pain is getting worse. "Maybe we can get rid of that IV today," Ann tells him, smiling. He grunts. "Maybe I can get rid of this hospital," he says. And he smiles too, grimly. After taking her leave, Ann tells me in the hall, "That's the longest sentence I've ever heard him say."

Farther down the hall an elderly man with cancer tattooed throughout his body lies in pain. He has just been admitted, the paperwork still unfinished, and none of the staff has ever met him or his family before. The man is confused, sedated, wincing in pain with moans between his disconnected words. "It's one of the problems with cancer treatment now," Ann says. "Since the docs do so much chemotherapy in their offices these days, we often don't see the patients here until they're really sick." She makes a note on the small pad in her pocket, to let the man's physician know about his discomfort, and to call the family.

Ellen Sandburg is back, to Ann's surprise. Ellen, a pretty and pale woman in her late thirties, was sent home from the hospital a few days earlier after another round of medication. Her ovarian cancer has spread into her lungs.

Since she went home Ellen has been dizzy and too nauseated to eat. Her white blood count, a measure of the
body's ability to fight infection, is 300—normal counts
are in the 4000 to 10,000 range. Her platelets, which help
in blood clotting, are less than a fifth of normal. She has
a nosebleed while she speaks to Ann. They chat about
her nausea, what kind of food she might be able to hold
down.

A smiling, obese woman rides by on a stretcher on her
way to the floor below for her daily radiation treatment.

Ann makes her phone calls. She talks one physician
into ordering a large dose of morphine for the elderly
man in so much pain. She calls out to a nurse walking
by, and within a few moments the bag of medication is
hung over the man's head, dripping into the IV tube in
his forearm, enough to put him to sleep in peace. She
tries to call his family, but no one answers.

On another phone in the square of desks a social worker
talks. He is telling a colleague about one of his patients,
a middle-aged woman, and her husband. "She told me
they have a suicide pact in case she's too sick to go home
from the hospital," he murmurs. He wonders about a
court order to protect her "from herself." His voice drops
to a whisper, concerned, bent over the sheaf of papers
in front of him.

A half-hour later, the nurse who fetched the medication waits for Ann to hang up the phone and then informs
her that the elderly man has died. Ann sighs. "Shoot."
It's Monday. She grabs the resident as he walks by, a tall,
bearded, quiet man looking as if he wished he had something to do. She tells him to go declare death. This resident has worked on this ward only a few days. Before
he closes the door of the man's room behind him, he
glances both ways as though to duck in without being
seen.

Lily and her husband arrive at the desk. Lily is here

for five days of medication to battle her ovarian cancer. Everyone in view calls a greeting to her. She smiles and kisses her tall, bald husband goodbye. He sets the overnight bag on the floor beside her and mournfully retreats the way they came. "Got any singles?" she asks Ann. "Not today, Lily, we're busy," she answers. "Oh, heck. Well, any doubles without anyone in them? Give me one of those; maybe I'll get lucky." She catches the eye of a nurse passing by with a tray of syringes. "It's hard to make cheerful conversation when you're not feeling cheerful," she tells her cheerfully.

A man arrives, hurried and anxious. He is unsure of himself. Finally, he asks the nurse standing next to Ann where to find a certain patient. Ann's head comes up, and she and the nurse glance at each other. This is the son of the man who just died. By the corner of the desk Ann puts her hand on the man's arm and says, "Your father passed away a short while ago." She speaks slowly, to give him time to hear the words. "We tried to call you. I'm sorry."

E VERY LITTLE ODD ACHE, CRAMP, TENSION; EACH SORE throat, swollen gland, headache; a sudden pain when you reach for something on a shelf, a morning lethargy, an unexpected reluctance: all these whisper *cancer*. Sings a poet: "As I was going up the stair, I met a man who wasn't there. . . ." Cancer climbs onto your back like a monkey, unseen; it digs in its claws when you try to run. The weighing down, the heaviness of suspicion, lingers long after we're told it's gone away.

We are worried. One survey of people's knowledge of cancer revealed a fair fraction of folks who believe that 50 to 100 percent of us will get cancer. We are cautioned against such a phobia, not to let the fear take hold and oppress us, but the truth is that millions of us will get cancer, one of every four, and most of us who get it will eventually die from it. This is a disease in which living is called a "clinical benefit" of the treatment, and success is measured in small segments of time during which the person hasn't died. It lends itself a little too easily to metaphors of psychic pain and disorganization, analogies of cultural disruption and personal failure. Cancer has been with us for a long time.

What do we know? Not much—peculiar facts. We know that cancer of the tongue is fairly common among men in Bombay but rare among the Maori tribes of New Zealand—and that if a Maori moves to Bombay, he faces a higher risk of tongue cancer in the future. Eskimo tribes and the people of Malta are having more cancer of the pharynx these days; nuns have a high rate of breast cancer. We know that two people with an identical cancer may respond in completely different ways to medical treatment. Gleeful clusters of cells, like schools of fish, can swim through the blood and spinal fluid to the shores of a new world. We really don't know very much about our friend cancer.

But we do have a sprawling mass of information, a mass that can remind us uncomfortably of a tumor. In the medical library near my home, in the ceiling-high stacks of magazines and journals arranged alphabetically, an entire bookcase a room wide is dedicated to periodicals beginning with the word "cancer." This is but a fraction. Who can read all this? Researchers make a living just writing reviews of other researchers' work, compiling it, organizing it, trying to make some sense out of it. Interesting what the researchers have found necessary to study: I've come across not one, not two, but dozens of scholarly and quite serious pieces devoted to proving that people with cancer tend to get depressed.

ONE OF THE QUALITIES COMMON TO CANCER SPECIALISTS is an immediate and intense dislike for what they call "quackery," alternative theories of cancer cause and cure. These phony medicine men and slick-talking practitioners, they tell us, are just out for money, preying on the helpless, the hopeless, the desperate. This dislike treads a thin line. Research, nice analytical research, continues to show that a variety of vitamins and certain foods can both help prevent and work to eradicate cancers—but ask your doctor about vitamin therapy. He is likely to be unimpressed. There is a dissonance here, ideas both contradictory and simultaneous. It is as though no truth can exist until it exists in the laboratory—and then it takes on a new name, a more complicated purpose and reason. There is more to the antagonism than simple philosophical territory. Cancer research is big business, one of the biggest in medicine—an industry. That's one source of the bristling. Even more is the nagging sense of a solution eluded, the taunts of boys against each other: after all those billions of dollars and decades of research, we don't know the cause, we can't prevent it, we don't know the cure, we can't even diagnose it much of the time until it's far advanced. Yes, there are cures—tumors go away, symptoms disappear, people climb out of their beds and walk home. But we don't always know where the cure comes from, for the untreated are cured sometimes as well. Knowing so little about the thing itself, having so much information and so little understanding, desperate to classify and define—perhaps it's a bit early to pat ourselves on the back for any apparent progress. Tumors go away by themselves, silent, enigmatic. We think the cancer has vacated because we persist in seeing it as separate from ourselves, discontinuous—and that is an easy thing to want to believe. Any assumption at all in the wake of small successes can be dangerous.

The researchers assume—need to believe—that the solutions have thus far evaded us because they lie in nothing simple, but are instead a complex and hieroglyphic mystery of the cell, a sequence decipherable only to a few initiated experts hoping to stumble across the key. Therefore, the mounds of impenetrable chemistry and the mountains of repeated trials and cautious hypotheses continue to grow. The scramble for grant money and fellowships can partly explain away the supercilious articles on depression. But it's that fear of failure that irritates the researchers most. Meanwhile, these Andean piles have gained us—what? All but the last step of the journey? Perhaps nothing much at all. For every ten women who get ovarian cancer, eight will die in less than five years, a fact that hasn't changed in three decades.

I'VE SEEN A NUMBER OF PEOPLE DIE OF CANCER—SOME quickly, some slowly. I've seen a few live with it too, some seem even to shake the monkey off. But all have to confront it, sooner or later, no matter how hard or delayed the confrontation, and pick a strategy. What can you do with a tumor curled up to your belly? Embrace it or be rid of it—and much of the "alternative" therapy for cancer claims the true key lies in some combination of the two. To embrace your tumor is to acknowledge its life, to say, as one might to a cat prowling uninvited in the pantry, yes, you are whole, you have desires, but you cannot satisfy them here. Be gone, cat, and take your smile with you.

Strike first with the knife. Cancers often form along particular organs, billowing up the side of the liver, stomach, kidney, or brain. Unfortunately, they curl up tightly to things we'd rather not part with. This loss is the first one; others follow.

One reaction people have when they discover they have cancer is a kind of revulsion, a disgust at this fecund birth inside them. To have it cut away can be a relief and a benevolence. The knife slides in and cuts it away, and that only validates its alien identity, something apart and not of you. If it cuddles up so close that part of you pulls away with it, well—perhaps that's best. Contamination, then, cutting your slack a little, but coming away from it clean.

Other cancers are "inoperable." A chilling word, with its intimations of negative outcomes and poor feedback mechanisms. Inoperable tumors are of three types, generally: those which spread so far and wide, hither and yon across the interior, that too little of you would be left after cutting; those which wind around delicate structures not meant to be sliced, such as the frontal lobe of the brain; and cancers of the blood and bone marrow, which aren't isolated tumors at all.

Surgery, drugs, and radiation are put together to form combination therapies. Every week the journals, in their proliferation, print new articles comparing one combination therapy to another, one approach to another, for the hundreds of different diseases called "cancer." If one works this well, perhaps another will work better, perhaps to add this drug, to cut sooner, to do radiation treatments longer. The physician in charge must manage the possibilities, the mathematics, by reading the research and asking around.

Radiation kills cells, shrinks them up like the feet of the wicked witch after Dorothy's house fell on her. Radiation can completely destroy some tumors and reduce the size of others, so even in terminal cases it may be used for "palliation"—to reduce pressure for relief from pain.

Several kinds of brain tumors, especially tumors that have spread from another site, are treated in part by radiation. At the beginning, the line of radiation is demarcated on the outside of the skull. It is drawn in indelible ink, so that each day the hot beam will fall on the same corner. The treatments last mere moments, unseen, unheard flashes of heat that one can hardly believe in, lying on the narow table, listening to the hum of the motor that moves the shield from the nugget of fire. As the days pass the hair falls out, the scalp grows tight and dry and wrinkled. The skin itches and can burn as though you had lain too long in the July sun. The black and purple lines of the field grow more prominent as the skull grows bald.

I REMEMBER TWO PEOPLE WHO SHARED A KIND OF TUMOR and a kind of treatment, with little else in common. Helen, still in her forties, was a thin, stately woman who was the matriarch of a large, close-knit family. She and her husband were deaf and mute and communicated only with sign language. Their children spoke, but not to members of the family. Sometimes five people would gather in Helen's room, taking seats on the windowsill and in her wheelchair, and talk animatedly, laughing, bearing news: all in silence, hands shooting through the air like comets. I felt inadequate, interrupting the commotion, stupid and illiterate.

Helen's son taught me to say a few words: bedpan, pain, eat, love, sleep. She took her pain medication without comment, and I would wonder whether she was stoic or simply so used to silence that even her pain was to be suffered without sound.

Radiation to her brain tumor made her sick to her stomach and very weak. She rapidly lost weight. After a week of treatments, she was bald and her face flaked in dry patches like peeling paint. The tumor was not responding, not shrinking; she was not going to get well.

Just a few days before she died, she asked me to put her on the commode, a bedside toilet. The morphine she had swallowed every few hours for weeks made her constipated most of the time. When I returned fifteen minutes later to help her back to bed, she was crying. I'd never seen her cry. As I put my arms under hers to ease the few steps, she collapsed, her thin legs suddenly too tired to hold her, and she dropped tears on my arm. Not a sound passed from her.

During these same weeks, Charlie stayed in a room down the hall. He was much older than Helen, without a family, and far from silent. He suffered the indignity of the cancer as he continued to suffer the other indignities life had pressed upon him: two fingers were missing from one hand, and one eye was false. He told his miseries to any who walked in—and sometimes by—his door.

The radiation flayed Charlie's skin and hair off his skull in bright red stripes. A few days after the treatments had begun he had an allergic reaction to a medication and his whole body turned lobster-red; it was covered with spots and itched without respite—itched hot, he told me, so that he felt himself burning up in the pricking of many tiny needles. I began bathing him with cold, wet towels. They would get warm in a few minutes; I would have to change the water to keep it cool. He was exhaling the heat as though he'd taken the radiation in and become a fuel source.

"I want to die," he would announce to each and all. The socket of his missing eye was irritated and draining; he'd had to take the globe out and store it in his drawer, a last indignity. Once he looked at me with the one good eye, the other a sunken fold, and said, "Kill me." It was a peremptory demand. He needn't have sought assistance. The cancer killed Charlie a few days later.

Little jars of radiation can be put inside a person. They can be sewn into the skin above the tumor, swallowed or breathed, gently inserted in a vagina. During the time of such treatments, the patient is dangerous, a reactor. He or she is confined to bed, treated with gloves, talked to from a distance. The heat of the radiation meets the metabolic heat of an erupting tumor, and the two energies explode, canceling each other out, sometimes taking the whole world with them.

Every war has a weapon of particular horror. In World War I it was mustard gas, the chemical that kills by burning, inside and out, sometimes quickly and sometimes not. It exfoliates mucus membranes the way napalm peels off palm tree's bark. Doctors treating mustard gas victims noted, in passing, that they had very low white blood counts and their bone marrow production was slowed. Since leukemia is an overgrowth of white cells, the physicians made an astute connection and found a silver lining to the war. Medicine often advances during war, after all; there is nothing like disaster to create human laboratories. Modern chemotherapy was, in a very real sense, the contribution of World War I. In a modified form, mustard gas is still being used against leukemia and lymph cancers.

Cancer cells have two particular characteristics: they are usually fast and they are always primitive. They multiply in a haphazard, unproductive way, fast and faster. They are called "nondifferentiated" because they have no special function; cancer cells don't grow up to be skin cells or liver cells or nerve cells. They live only to reproduce again, take up more space. Cancer cells are usually bigger than normal cells, and they are shaped differently, amorphous. But they are also different from each other, each harking to a different call. No beehive here, no orderly rows or camps of cells all neatly tucked in together like logs in a log house. These queer birds go their own way, laughing, making ragged sheets and tangled nests of cells. Most disturbing of all, they seem to thrive on trouble, growing in circumstances that would kill normal cells. In fact, abnormal conditions can speed the growth of tumors, and the bigger they get, the hungrier they are.

A tumor is called a neoplasm—a growth that serves no function living at the expense of the host. A parasite. The roots of the word "neoplasm" are a "thing recently formed," and such is the tumor: it grows and changes so quickly it is always new, always being formed. Anticancer drugs are properly called "antineoplastics," but in the business people call them "chemotherapy." The idea of drug therapy in cancer is that a fast-growing cell can be killed by interfering with any of its several phases of growth; since a tumor has any number of cells in different phases of growth at any time, drugs that attack in several different phases are best. Combinations of drugs can serve the same purpose. Cancer drugs are only slightly selective for their target; they hit all fast-growing cells—our hair, stomach and intestinal linings, and skin. The "margin of safety is often very narrow," says one textbook calmly. Ellen Sandburg is suffering her nausea, weakness, and nosebleeds not from the cancer but from the chemotherapy; it has weakened her to a dangerous state. Chemotherapy is like weeding a wheat field by walking through it with a sickle mowing down whole swaths of grain.

Each cancer drug has a certain "kill rate." A chemical with an 80 percent kill rate generally kills 80 percent of the cancer cells with each dose. This accomplishes a kind of exponential decline over time, a reverse of the startling exponential growth of the disease. Physicians design drug regimens that will, it is hoped, kill as many cancer cells as possible as quickly as possible without killing the host. The patient is the village that must be destroyed in order to be saved. Methotrexate is a drug used in the treatment of several types of cancer. When it is given in high doses,

severe kidney and liver damage can occur. To counter-
mand the potentially fatal effects of methotrexate, it is
followed several hours later by another drug called leucovorin, which bumps the methotrexate off the cells. This
is called the "leucovorin rescue." If rescue is delayed too
long or the doses are too low, the damage from the methotrexate can be permanent.

Drugs are given once a week, or for several days at a
time every few weeks, or every day—whatever combination appears most likely to work. Patients are resigned
to six months, twelve months, two years—even longer in
some cases—of side effects. Will your hair fall out? Will
you vomit till your stomach seems to hang outside your
mouth? There's only one way to tell. Will the drugs kill
the particular cells of your particular tumor? There's only
one way to tell, and time is a-wasting.

I'm sure the cancer specialists are impatient with all my
gloom by now. After all, millions of people are walking
around who "beat" cancer: 2 million according to the
National Institute of Health; 3 million according to the
American Cancer Society. How many hidden mastectomies, colostomies, ileostomies, and hysterectomies do you
pass in the bank and the grocery store every day? Pessi-
mism about cancer treatment is one side of a line that
falls like a sharp shadow through the ward: either you
live or you die.

"I WAS A REAL DIFFICULT PATIENT. MY SURGEON STRUG-
gled with me a lot; I was real angry, real nasty to that
poor man, and he's just this very nice, very quiet type. I
was taking things out on him. I was *real* angry. Because
you go through life and you see a lot of people who just
trash their bodies, could care less about their health—

and it just didn't seem fair, and there was an awful lot of anger. And I think that carried me through sometimes —it gave me something to fight *with*."

Words and pictures fail to describe clearly a woman like Evelyn Marley. In all fairness, to get a sense of Evelyn one must sit on her sofa by the fireplace listening to the continual chatter and buzz of the finches in the row of cages behind you, watching Evelyn move and smile and laugh, throw her head back in a giggle and wave her hands around as she struggles to get a point across. Evelyn is very pretty, blond, round, and bright-cheeked, and she's happy.

Five years ago, when she was twenty-five, Evelyn found a lump in her right breast. She went on a scheduled vacation without seeing her doctor. "In the back of my mind I was really conscious of the change. The tumor really did grow in those two weeks. I could feel the pressure of it, feel the change. I knew that it was malignant." She returned from the beach and soon found herself topless in front of an internist she'd never met before, a cancer specialist. "He drew a circle around it so another doctor could look at it, and then he told me it was cancer, by feeling it, without a biopsy. I wasn't ready to hear that. He didn't say, 'What do you think about that? Do you have anyone to drive you home? Can you *stand up?*' I mean, it's like he didn't realize—he couldn't have hit me harder if he'd knocked me over. The man had absolutely no empathy or concern. He just said, 'It's malignant and it's going to have to be removed.' And just sent me out."

Evelyn thinks now, as she's thought about that moment many times, and adds, "Maybe I wanted them to ease me into it. And I needed them to say, 'But this doesn't mean you're going to be dead.' They forget about everything you read about cancer in the paper. They can take out the word 'cancer' and put in the word 'death.' It's almost synonymous. Some bad press there."

She was sent for a mammography, an x-ray test of the breast tissues that can spot a tumor too small to feel. A second lump was found in the right breast, and several small lumps were also found in the left breast. At the time, five years ago, it was still routine procedure to do an amputation of the breast—a mastectomy—on the surgical table as soon as the lump was found to be malignant. The patient didn't wake from anesthesia first; the results were always a surprise. The consent forms given to potential breast cancer victims included permission to do complete mastectomies before the diagnosis of cancer was confirmed. Evelyn refused to sign. "They pressured me —they came back in my room and asked me if I fully understood. Now I know why they strap you to those gurneys—I'd have rather been anywhere but there." She wanted to investigate alternatives, tried to round up enough money to go to a Mexican clinic, to get some laetrile. She agreed to a biopsy, only, on each breast. Both were malignant. "I was really struggling for time to make up my own decisions; they were push, push, push. Once they did the biopsy, that was it—you're going in tomorrow. All the time in my heart I knew that if I wanted to live I probably did need to have the surgeries. And I did have the option to keep the left breast and have radiation, but radiation was too frightening to me."

A few weeks after the biopsies, with no clear alternative available, Evelyn had a modified radical mastectomy on her right breast, in which the breast and most of the nearby lymph nodes were removed. A week later she had a simple mastectomy on the left, in which only the breast was removed. But her shocks weren't over. As she began to eat her first meal after the second surgery, a doctor she had never met came into her hospital room. He'd been asked to consult on her case by her regular doctor. "He came into my room and told me it was a good thing my meal was cold because it would wait," Evelyn remembers, and one still sees the anger in her smile. "He informed me I had some real problems, and he thought a year and a half to two years of chemotherapy would be appropriate, and I really should consider having a complete hysterectomy. I was twenty-five years old. I had not had any children, and the last month had been real fun. This man talking—and not even 'How are you?' or 'Are you feeling okay?' None of the formalities. I informed him that they couldn't continue to carve me up like I was a bar of soap, and I had some rights and some things to think about." She recently went over her medical records with a new physician. "I'm really incensed about this now, because in my file was this asshole's letter about me, and he was so biased! The letter said 'This angry, hostile young woman.' He even called me unfortunate! He felt really sorry for me, and then he thanked the doctor for the referral."

She began chemotherapy, once a week for a year and a half. She lost her job because of missing so much work, and she was evicted from her house when she couldn't pay the rent. She had no insurance, and she didn't qualify for welfare.

By this time in her treatment, Evelyn was marked as angry. She demanded the right to have a bottle of vitamins by her bedside during her treatments. "It may sound really strange," she says now, "but I was thinking about some of the reasons why I was able to pull through, and it's because I was able to establish a very, very small element of control. I had really strong fears about chemotherapy. Unless you're knowledgeable, all you hear about are the people who died. And it's not always clear whether they died from the disease or the treatment. Now I know it's questionable still. It was as if I was being a disobedient child."

"The first time the bandages were off, the showers were horrible. I hated showers. It was a straight shot down, and no matter how thin I was, my stomach just stuck out huge. You have this protective bandage on—they bandage you up so much it almost looks as if you have breasts. I didn't have much trouble looking at it after the surgery, I guess, because I'd never seen anything like it. It was when it was healed and it still didn't look good . . ."

Evelyn was given a prescription for breast prostheses, the artificial pads worn inside a bra to give shape after mastectomies. "I can remember putting them gently back in the box, being so careful with them. Then after a while, I remember throwing them at my boyfriend, putting one on the dog's head—it had a real cone shape, made him look like a little Trojan warrior. It sounds strange. I had to learn to laugh at them; I had to learn to laugh at myself. I remember walking through a crowd one time and having my bra unhook." The pads just fell out. One of her boyfriend's friends asked her curiously: "How do you know which way to put your clothes on?" She retorted: "How do *you?*"

Two years after her original surgeries, Evelyn went in for reconstruction, a process she initiated and carried through on her own. Reconstruction of the breasts is a plastic surgery technique that implants an artificial prosthesis in the chest wall to "pad out" the flattened area in a semblance of breasts. Later on, if only one breast has been removed, a nipple can be grafted onto the new breast from the healthy nipple. In some cases, the nipple is "rescued" from the amputated breast and "banked" in the groin, like an image from some erotic Freudian dream, where it grows normally until the time is right to reimplant it on the new breast. This last procedure is losing popularity, though, because in some cases the nipple has carried the cancer with it to the reconstructed area. Reconstruction is erratically successful; implants can slip, migrate, and often don't have a normal shape. Evelyn pats her blouse and says, "This one's flat, and this one's a little rounder. They don't look like breasts. I went through the same process of standing in the shower and being almost hysterical. I called my doctor and said, 'What did you do to me?' I was terribly disappointed, because it wasn't perfect. There were still scars. I *knew* there would be scars. I guess in my mind's eye I was thinking he was going to give me a really good approximation of what my breasts had been, and he couldn't. When I get in the shower now, I at least have some kind of shape."

She lives in a large, airy house with a new roommate; she has a new boyfriend; she has a new job. Evelyn is getting her master's degree in social work; she wants to work with physicians, teach them a "better way to take care of people." There is still a question of whether she should have children, because the hormones involved in pregnancy have the potential to trigger a tumor again. She laughs and laughs, telling stories, awful stories, about her experience. She laughs and gets tears in her eyes and looks intently at me, still angry. "A woman saw me later and said, 'I never thought you'd make it—you were so angry.' I guess the question is, 'What is a healthy response?'"

"**T**HE RELATIONSHIP BETWEEN PAIN AND THE EMOTIONAL state of the cancer patient must be clearly recognized. Pain may provide a means for the cancer patient to express anguish." So says a recent cancer textbook. But the pain may be a source of the anguish being expressed. More theories again. About 60 to 80 percent of patients hospitalized with advanced cancer have severe pain. Pain can be the first warning, that original nagging ache—and it can withhold its presence until the end. The growing tumors press on nerves and blood vessels and other parts of you; joints stiffen, and swollen and inflamed tissue surrounds them. Cancer pain has a unique quality to the suffering; it is constant, unrelenting, unrelieved. It fades and brightens, tacks and jibes, but never—not even in sleep—does it disappear. Not unless that which digs its thumbs in is removed.

The cancer patient and the burn patient have much in common. Both have been visited by devastation. Both have lost much that was dear. Both suffer quantities of pain, buckets of it, and both are given more pain for their trouble. The burn patient quivers while the dressings are changed; the cancer patient vomits and frays. Lucky, both, that research is so diligently ferreting out whether their pain is real, whether they might not be better given a tranquilizer or antidepressant than the cool wash of morphine.

Over fifteen years ago a textbook advocated ordering regular pain medication for cancer patients, but this is still uncommon. Many studies have shown that both physicians and nurses tend to give too little medication too infrequently to relieve pain in cancer patients. In some cases physicians say they will even decrease the dose or use a placebo when a patient's complaints of pain continue. Only one reason is consistently given by these health professionals eager to give the best of care: the possibility of addiction. Like burn pain, the chronic pain of cancer absorbs the drug, drinking it in, and narcotics can give pain relief without any sensation of a narcotic high, a muted norm. But that straight-laced anxiety remains, almost a contempt. We become mothers, overly concerned with doing the right thing, always searching the patient for that successful adjustment to the sick role, the surrender to sorrow. So do we look beneath the promised pain and the sick person's suffering for expressions of anguish, symptoms of depression, an objective measurement. So do we protect him from an imaginary, future shame.

What seems forgotten is how addiction often develops. Addiction is a product of preoccupation, of obsession. In pain, unable to think of anything else, counting the minutes until the next dose will be permitted—and then having to ask, always having to ask because the drug has been ordered on an "as necessary" basis by the physician and so never makes it on the nurse's schedule of drugs to be given at certain times—here is a person already psychologically addicted, already humiliated. He can think of nothing *but* his pain and its relief; he is already defeated and at our mercy. Here is a junkie.

This is what I must do when my cancer patient asks for a dose of narcotic. I find the physician's order and check the dose allowed, the frequency, and when she last received it. If the time is right, I make sure the order is current—sometimes narcotic orders must be renewed every week or two. Then I find the keys, for narcotics are locked up, and locked again. I find the room, the cart of medication or the drawer, and the bin of narcotics all locked. I find the narcotic book, and in the book I find the line for the particular medication (say, Demerol, a synthetic narcotic, in 50 milligram doses). I pull out the box of Demerol vials or pills, check the dose, and check the number. The book says twenty-four should be left. Are there twenty-four? Yes. So I take one, write the patient's name, her room number, her physician, my name, the dose, the date, the time, and how many vials are left. I am careful to lock up. Then she gets her shot. If when I count the medicine there are too few to match the book or, at the end of the day, if a narcotic is unaccounted for, I have to write an incident report, describing the entire procedure. If I draw the medicine up and go to her room and she's changed her mind, doesn't want it—or if I drop the pill on the floor—I have to find another nurse. Together we pour the medicine down the toilet and both of us sign the book—"narcotic wasted." At the beginning and end of each shift, two nurses count every single dose of every narcotic left.

All this rigmarole is because narcotics are categorized as "controlled substances." Any drug that has the potential for causing addiction is handled in this way, and people are very, very chary about them. Pharmacies and houses are robbed for these drugs; nurses who pocket a few will lose their licenses. As a student nurse years ago I was watching a throat surgery. I saw the circulating nurse sign out a vial of cocaine, used to numb the throat and stop the bleeding, and then drop the vial in her pocket rather than lay it with the other medications. I asked her why she handled it that way and she rather impolitely told me that a few narcotics had recently been missing; in this way she could keep an eye on it. Much to my surprise, my instructor took me aside hours later and told me I'd been reported for showing "undue curiosity" about the cocaine. The nurse wondered if I was a thief. Whenever something comes up short, all the nurses—since it is only nurses who carry keys—take a breath and hold it, hoping they won't be accused.

All this is to keep those drugs which make us feel good in the proper hands—that is, out of the hands of people who would take them just to feel good. That is not permitted, and I am charged with being sure that my patients, cancer or no, aren't taking them for that reason either.

The English, in that civilized way of English writers, tell us in the medical journals that heroin is the best cure for pain in cancer, unexcelled, a grace. In this country we give morphine, methadone, aspirin, and various synthetic drugs for cancer pain and take up space in American journals with studies trying to show that all these are just as good as heroin. A controversy, a tempest fought away from the bedside. I'm just waiting for my pill, says the patient.

Methadone is an interesting drug. It is a narcotic used most often to treat heroin addicts in detoxification programs, but more and more often for cancer. Methadone is less likely to cause either sedation or euphoria than heroin and morphine, and once a person has become tolerant of a certain dose, taking other narcotics has little effect. Methadone is also addictive. A person can be switched from heroin addiction to methadone addiction in a few weeks; the result is still a junkie, but one with a legal habit who will get little joy from other narcotics—and thus little motivation to take them. Methadone has been used to treat cancer patients more frequently in the last few years partly because it can be taken by mouth rather than being injected—and partly because of its joylessness. The artificial tranquility of heroin and morphine is exactly what gives them "potential for abuse." Never mind that terminally ill patients who are given either drug say they experience little pleasure from them—the intensity and constancy of the pain seem to "absorb" pleasure for cancer patients in the same way they do for burn patients. We are protecting them from the *possibility* of pleasure, of dreamy rest, of absence and release. The pain, it seems, (once we admit it exists) can be permitted to be erased, but not replaced.

The trick with methadone is that its worth depends on keeping a steady level in the bloodstream. Methadone must be given regularly, around the clock, never late or forgotten. If a person is getting too much, you can't skip a dose and catch up; you must reduce the amount of every dose and keep giving it. Methadone is the acid test of cancer nursing: pay proper attention and you can help free a person from pain; grow absentminded, forget your homework, and you may as well have done nothing at all. The real secret to controlling pain is to stop the perception of pain before it begins—in the nerve cells, across the synapses, in consciousness.

The Food and Drug Administration recently approved a new drug called naltrexone. It is an opoid antagonist —its only purpose is to block the effects of such drugs as opium, morphine, and, incidentally, methadone. Naltrexone will be used to treat recovering addicts, including methadone addicts, in the same way and for the same reason that methadone has been used to treat heroin addicts. Inordinate and dangerous pleasure is traded for ordinary life, and then that is made addictive; with methadone, even the routine lack of euphoria becomes essential.

Perhaps one reason pain medication has been so badly managed is that it "requires the explicit or at least tacit admission that the disease is incurable." I wonder, watching nurses avoid certain rooms, hearing the bad jokes of the residents and the detached, arm's-length language of the physicians: do we blame them, these patients? If a man who has smoked two packs of cigarettes a day for thirty years finds himself dying of lung cancer, perhaps he should die in pain. He has brought this on himself, and we know it—and he knows we know it. The table turns, and he also knows, as do we, that there's nothing that can be done. This shared and guilty knowledge isn't enough: it is not all right, not to be given, that his death be pain-free. This is his punishment.

Recent years have seen a proliferation of books about the "cancer personality," treatises that aim to connect behavior and character with disease. The connection is not a new one, and neither are the conclusions of the authors. Sin, guilt, and abuse and misuse of the body we are given at birth, the maltreatment we receive from the world— all are accused of the genesis of disease. Where does cancer come from, this illness that lends itself too easily to metaphor? Do we repress anger and grow tumors instead, sorrow in secret until our cells explode in a rage of compensation? Do we give cancer to each other, one to one, the way we pass out moods and ideas? Do we sit like blood brothers slitting fingertips and pressing the fluid together, sealing fate?

"They made me feel guilty," says Evelyn Marley about the books she bought after her diagnosis. "They made me feel as if I'd wanted to get cancer." Cancer patients are often ashamed, self-conscious, chagrined at the weak character that allowed them to succumb to a "lifestyle" illness. What a cruel kind of comfort to offer, after the fact. Even the patient is a judge.

S EVERAL MONTHS AGO THE NURSING CENTER WHERE I worked admitted a woman in her sixties who was dying of cancer of the neck. She knew she was dying; her family brought with her suitcase a favorite armchair, a pile of books, a small television, and several plants. She moved into the only room then available, the single room with a private bath usually reserved for isolation cases. She took the seclusion and created her own death from it.

The woman had had a permanent tracheostomy as part of the cancer treatment, and she was left unable to speak. She refused to learn the methods by which such people can regain a form of speech. In fact, she refused everything: she refused to be bathed, to have the tracheostomy cleaned or bandaged, to have the room cleaned, the wastebaskets emptied. Her wound drained mucus, which she wiped away with tissues; the pile of tissues accumulated. She couldn't speak, wouldn't try; often she would refuse even to write a note. She wouldn't look us in the eye, and when we came in the room, she would cover her neck (it was only a small hole, a slight scar to our jaded eyes) with her hands and turn away. The room smelled; she smelled. We were torn between the desire to let her have the death of her choosing, the privacy she craved, and our own need to care for her, clean her up, and cheer the dark corners of the room.

I know many physicians and nurses who would have treated her for the obvious depression and withdrawal with tranquilizers and antidepressants and would have given physical care even if it meant sedating her. We chose the decision of inaction, and it was hard. A few things were done, trash taken out and floors mopped, and we left her alone. The room was equipped with a closed-circuit television, and I still don't know if she realized that we could watch her from the distance of the nurse's desk.

In the last days before she died she lay for many hours with hardly a movement. We had several false alarms of death, only to look closer and see her head turn a fraction, see her sigh. I do not know and never will whether she died a good death or a bad one—whether she punished herself for her illness and was rewarded with atonement, or whether she punished herself and found no reward at all. For all I know, and it isn't much, she chose a healthy and thoughtful death, making manifest without need for polite explanations the isolation of all who are dying.

THIS JUDGMENT IS EVERYWHERE. A PARTICULAR CANCER, uncommon, begins in the blood vessels. The first symptom is usually purple or dark-brown spots on the toes and legs. For decades this cancer has been a footnote, an oddity—until recently. Now people who had spent their professional lives without seeing this disease have become experts in its diagnosis and treatment. The cancer is Kaposi's sarcoma, and it is associated with AIDS.

Acquired immune deficiency syndrome—AIDS—is both literally and metaphorically the cancer that can be caught. It is the penultimate surrender of the ill to the illness, an involuntary succumbing, a giving up. The invisible hostility of the world becomes visible, palpable, apocalyptic.

Infectious diseases attack the various cells of the body, the way meningitis got a hold on Aaron and dug in its toes. The army of one attacks the army of the other, and the symptoms that follow are simple and old-fashioned war, filled with skirmishes and a variety of tactics. Losses are felt on both sides, and eventually one wins out. But AIDS, whatever causes it, whatever creates it or begins it—be it virus or a new molecule altogether or nothing at all—whatever AIDS is, it has a new strategy. AIDS is the new first-strike weapon, the Trident submarine of illnesses. Forget the old method of hand-to-hand combat, soldier to soldier. AIDS blows up the weapons, bombs the munition dumps, and lays siege. Soon, very soon, the environment does its work for it, because the body can no longer battle any bug, any germ, at all.

AIDS patients fight themselves as well, becoming allergic to their own cells. They catch rare diseases, infectious diseases such as cryptosporidiosis, which had only six recorded cases from 1976 to 1981 worldwide and then fourteen cases in gay men alone in the next year. AIDS patients get ill from bugs that don't bother anyone else; they get thrush, a cottage cheese-like yeast infection of the mouth, and so on. A particular pneumonia, *Pneumocystis carinii*, preys on AIDS patients, a pneumonia rarely seen in anyone else. The whole idea of an opportunistic infection has taken on new meaning because of AIDS, no longer confined to the virulent and mean. It is as though a whole new generation of formerly friendly organisms has seen the light.

Everything that happens to AIDS patients—but to a more controlled, more specific degree—happens to cancer patients who are given immunosuppressive drugs and to kidney transplant recipients who take steroids. Like the strike of lightning that burns off the face, it is not a highly contagious destiny, but a strangely selective one.

All of the sick are expatriates, forever homesick. The victims of AIDS are also exiled—their alienation is taken a step beyond mere decay. They die in isolation rooms, attended by the masked and gloved, who are scared behind their costumes. AIDS has become an agent of right and wrong, made so by the not-sick, but no amount of penance and retribution will influence its course. Kaposi's sarcoma is itself evolving, finding new stones to step on. In increasing numbers Kaposi's is being reported in kidney transplant patients, in people with other cancers who get immunosuppressive therapy, in other groups of people receiving the boon of medicine. Its lesions are spreading, appearing on the gums, the rectum, the intestine—where they may hemorrhage until a person bleeds to death. And how is it treated? With radiation, with chemotherapy.

R ICHARD IS A PHYSICIAN'S ASSISTANT IN A CLINIC WHERE I volunteer on occasion. We were friendly acquaintances when we decided to split the cost of Spanish lessons, given by a Panamanian nurse named Hilda. She would not allow us to speak English during lessons, and even in our most fumbling ignorance we were forced to search for a way to say what we wanted to say.

One morning, before lessons began, Richard turned to me. In forbidden English he said, "They want to do a radical neck on me. I have metastatic cancer." I knew immediately who "they" were, and I knew what a "radical neck"—a complex and mutilating surgery on the throat —would mean. Richard is 35 years old, strong, vigorous, and quick to laugh. He was planning to leave for three weeks of wilderness hiking when he discovered the nature of the lump on his neck.

Hilda arrived, and we spoke only Spanish. She is a nurse and teacher of no mean ability. She knew something was wrong, and that morning we learned *doloroso* for sorrowful and *miedo* for fear. With gestures, facial expressions, mismatched words, and tone, Richard, Hilda, and I talked about death. It was the first time he had been able to speak of it. "*Impuestos y muerte,*" she said, smiling. Taxes and death.

The physicians who work with Richard at the clinic, his fellow assistants, his friends who are nurses—Richard felt they turned from him with his diagnosis. He had his surgery, and it was less extensive than feared. He has his voice still, he has his throat, but the bushy bright-red beard is gone. He is glad I didn't "get weird" on him. His cancer has a survival rate of only five percent in five years. We speak Spanish haltingly, laughingly together. *Impuestos y muerte.*

FOUR WEEKS HAVE PASSED SINCE I LAST WALKED ROUNDS with Ann Burke. I'm back to talk to Lily while she has another round of chemotherapy. In those weeks Carl Burger went home and died. Ellen Sandburg died before she could go home. The young boy in the dark room died, too.

Lily is fifty-four years old and she looks forty. Part of it, I think, is the stylish ash-blonde wig she wears most of the time to cover her drug-bald head. She has a trim figure—she claims that during her first surgery for ovarian cancer, when most of the tumor was removed (called a "debulking" in the parlance of medicine), she was given a "tummy tuck" in the bargain. Lily comes to the hospital every four weeks for five days of chemotherapy. This is her fourth visit in a sequence of eight. She's not her usually jocular vivacious self today, but she is talkative nonetheless.

Talking takes her mind off the waves of nausea that sweep over her every time a new bottle of medication is started on her IV. "The first couple days aren't so bad, because your resistance is up," she says quietly, holding a basin under her chin in case she must throw up. "By the third day, though, you have your reactions right away, because by then you haven't had much to eat. At least I haven't—I can't eat their food. All I have to do is look at the menu to get sick to my stomach." Besides the nausea, Lily has numb fingers and toes, a side effect that lingers most of the time and may last up to a year after her last chemotherapy. "The weakness is the thing I notice at home," she says. "If I am very sparing and careful, I can get everything done, but I have to budget it like you do your money. Try not to do anything that takes a lot of muscle—like vacuuming. If I vacuum, it takes my strength for the whole day." These symptoms and, of course, the hair. Her wig is off now, since she spends these days in bed alone. Not a hair rises from her head, not even baby down, no stubble, no color. When the drugs are done and her hair returns, no one can predict what color, what texture it will be. A surprise, a midyear Christmas gift for Lily to look forward to in a few months.

She refuses visitors, including her husband, during the drug courses. "He worries and fusses and stews. He just doesn't need that stress—and neither do I." Lily sits up suddenly as another rush hits her stomach. Deep breathes for a moment, and then says, "You should never get can-

cer. I don't know if you can control it or not. I think all
your physical state is somewhat relative to your mental
state, and if you didn't get cancer, you'd get something.
I was a classic case of someone who was kind of asking
for it by not taking care of my mental problems." Before
her illness, Lily had a prolonged depression stemming
from strife in her marriage. She often uses it as an example, a version of before-cancer with which to compare
her ideas of after-cancer.

Lily emphasizes her attitude; she works it into every
conversation: "I'm going to beat it. I don't consider this
life-threatening. Other people die of cancer, but I won't."
She finds as many ways to say it as she can. "I won't put
up with depression, I'll tell you that. I'll get some professional help if I have to. Sometimes you feel like you have
no control, and now I realize that I *have* to get control
over it or I'll be sick again. That was my problem—I
thought there was some unsolvable problems, and I know
I could have solved those problems if I'd put my mind
to it. I thought maybe there was something wrong with
me."

W HAT IS CANCER IF NOT ITS COLLECTIVE SURVIVAL
rates? There is disease-free survival, with no sign
of cancer, and there is just plain survival, disease or not.
There is one-year survival, five-year survival, and ten-
year survival. Drug combinations are developed by comparing the survival rates of two groups of people getting
different combinations—but more on that in a minute.
Just to look at a few relevant rates is illustrative.

Lily is the one woman in seventy who will get ovarian
cancer. Seventy percent of *those* women will have an advanced stage of the disease by the time it is diagnosed.

Whether or not any one woman survives depends quite a lot on how much of the tumor is left in her belly after surgery. In those advanced cases, the cancer may have invaded the intestines, bladder, uterus, and the lining of the abdomen itself. What surgery takes then, in its de-bulking pride, is more than just an ovary. The surgeons are exhorted to be aggressive in their slicing.

What is left when the knife has come and gone is called residue, and if the residue is more than 2 centimeters large, the statistical chances for survival are slim. This is why ovarian cancer is fought sometimes with massive surgery, cutting away parts of the lower intestine and rectum, the bladder, and the entire reproductive system. Survival in any group of women with ovarian cancer varies from a low of 0 to 9 percent to a high of about 35 percent.

E VELYN HAS MORE COMPANY FOR HER MISSING AND RE-sculpted breasts than you may imagine. Breast cancer is the most common gynecological cancer in Western countries; one of every eleven women will get it. Breast cancer is also the leading cause of death in women between thirty-five and fifty-four years of age, and recent years have shown no improvement in survival rates.

After decades of blanket permission slips and routine radical mastectomies, women still aren't living any longer. All those breasts summarily consigned to the incinerator, to ashes, along with the lymph nodes and chest-wall muscles, and no help to the woman. Research has steadily and ploddingly shown that a less extensive surgery and even simply removal of the tumor alone can be as effective. At this time, several states require physicians to discuss all the medical options for breast cancer before a woman consents to surgery. But compare Evelyn's and

Lily's chances to those of a person with Hodgkin's disease. Ten years after diagnosis, 62 percent of the patients with this cancer are still alive. More than half—that *is* an improvement. It is Hodgkin's disease that is often pointed to and used to account for improved survival of cancer in general. Take almost any other kind of cancer, though, and the graphs look like steep and stumbling mountainsides down to the flat grass of near-zero as the first year, the second year, the fifth year roll by.

Statistics galore. Choosing a therapy is a choice between statistics, between which journals you read and who your colleagues are, between whose research you've read and how carefully you read it. Cancer specialists have pet regimens, and they change with time—seriously considered but always less than certain. Part of the problem is the unpredictability of response.

People whose tumors get smaller on a drug are considered "responders" to the drug—or rather, their tumor is a responder. There is no sure way to predict who in any group of people with similar cancers will be a responder. Nonresponders lose time, suffering through a regimen that does no good. But there's more: nonresponders are more easily weakened and debilitated by the chemotherapy. They are more susceptible to its damage at the same time that the tumor cells riding them are less so. Giving a nonresponder a heavy dose of chemotherapy can kill him or her. Do a few simple problems of research begin to appear?

Most chemotherapy research compares two groups of people receiving different combinations of drugs. The survival rates of the two groups are compared after some set period of time—say, six months and then again at one year or five years—for relative survival rates. The regimen given to the group with a higher survival rate is then considered the better drug. (Of course, the research will then be duplicated, replicated, and repeated, and individual physicians in the field will continue to give other combinations while the research is considered.) This comparison, because both groups will have responders and nonresponders in it—and one may have more than the other—is somewhat fallacious. A sidelight is the fact that in any one group the nonresponders on a drug therapy are most likely to die and thus skew the survival rate in their group against the whole group—even if the responders do very well.

A recent article pointed this out, without the usual dissembling. The physicians who wrote the study took a big chunk of chemotherapy research and restructured the kind of comparisons made to eliminate as much as possible the problem of nonresponders. They tried comparing survival rates between any group of people receiving a treatment and a matched group receiving no drug treatment at all. Their conclusion: "Most patients with cancer do not have tumors for which chemotherapy has been clearly demonstrated to be effective in prolonging life." Lest their work be thought too rough on well-meaning researchers, they added toward the end a consolation: "Investigators who were enthusiastic about their findings may have wanted to present their results in the best possible light."

The search continues. New drugs and old drugs looked at in new lights are always being considered for use against cancer. After studying a drug's effects on individual cells and then on animals, researchers have a sense of the drug's possible effect on tumors as well as its side effects on the patient. At this point a drug is introduced into phase I studies on humans with cancer. One is reminded of the cautionary tales about quackery when phase I studies are considered.

The purposes of such a study, say one drug handbook, are "to establish the toxicity of an investigational agent in humans, to establish a maximum tolerated dose in humans, and to determine an optimal dose and schedule. . . . Most patients participating in a phase I study have advanced metastatic cancer, with little or no chance of deriving benefit from known treatments, or have tumors that have become resistant to standard forms of therapy."

Put another way, a person dying of cancer, who is beyond the limited resources of traditional medicine, is offered a carrot on a stick, a last hope, a drug "still in the experimental stages" which may yet be the cure. As with organ transplants, with the middle-class heroes of the artificial heart, the dying can feel they have made a contribution, helped advance medical science—perhaps gain a few hours, perhaps lose a few. To establish toxicity in people weakened by terminal cancer is to find out how much of a drug will kill them. Just before that point, you see, is the "maximum tolerated dose."

The dying do make a contribution for their trouble. Unexpected side effects (or benefits) may appear in the course of a phase I study, and a clearer sense of dosage and timing as well as the effect of a drug on advanced, progressive cancer can be considered. These "fringe effects" are the only real purpose of a phase I study. Lives are not saved. It is just that people who are going to die anyway take the risks of the unknown.

If a drug "passes" its phase I study, either by virtue of making some dent in a tumor or improving a patient's response to other drugs, or similar drugs, and so on, it is given over to phase II testing. Patients in phase II trials have an active cancer that has some statistical chance of being cured by standard treatment. Phase II trials study the effect of a drug on fast-growing tumors and slow-growing tumors, as well as on specific types of cancer. Most experimental drugs—and there are many—never get this far.

Phase III is the last of the human experiments. A new drug is tested in patients who are being treated, and its effect (the survival rate, of course, and the size of tumors) is compared to that achieved by conventional drugs. After this all that is left is approval by the Food and Drug Administration.

Laetrile was dismissed as useless after it failed to improve the rate of survival of a group of terminally ill people. A 1985 article in the *New England Journal of Medicine* (which also published the laetrile study) came to the same conclusion about vitamin C. High doses of vitamin C did nothing to improve the survival of terminal cancer patients, and so it was declared "worthless."

This is the other problem with phase I studies. A new drug may be the cure for isolated, newly discovered tumors of a certain kind—but if it doesn't perform better than drugs already in hand on incurable patients, it can be rejected completely. Only if a researcher *wants* to use a drug, believes in it for whatever reason, will it pass to patients not yet deemed beyond hope. What manufacturer or researcher would really be happy to discover that vitamins can cure or prevent cancer? What glory then?

Informed consent is a problem in cancer research; in fact, it may be an impossibility. A signed consent form is no indication that informed consent has been obtained, and a person facing death from an incurable disease, offered one slim chance, may be the least capable adult to give a considered decision. So little time is left for consideration. Quite a number of people have written in the course of discussions about treatment of deformed babies that no one in the midst of a crisis is capable of making an informed decision. Surely facing one's own death constitutes a crisis at least as compelling as the care of one's defective child. But little has been written about the terminal cancer patient's freedom of choice, including the freedom to make what to some may be an irrational decision, that of turning away a possible miracle cure.

One of the experimental drugs, sooner or later, may very well be the cure, it is true, and that thin possibility gleams in the distance, a shining city.

If, in the course of a research study, the researcher in charge begins to suspect that the new drug in question is working poorly, he or she faces a dilemma: should the research be stopped ahead of schedule and should the patients be directed to other, possibly more efficacious treatments? Or should the research be continued to further knowledge? The same researcher, seeing that the drug seems to be working unexpectedly well, faces a different dilemma: should the results be proclaimed without finishing the study, thereby alerting other researchers to its potential? What if the researcher jumps the gun, wanting to present the results "in the best possible light"? The constrictures of research require a certain amount of conformity to custom, a certain detached approach, a way of keeping oneself out of the picture. Even when there may be nothing but grasping at straws, the articles must be written calmly, with a slight edge of optimism. Who better to choose for the future of an individual patient than the impartial researcher dedicated to finding a cure for cancer?

For all the distaste a phase I study leaves in the mouth, what else are we to do? Monoclonal antibodies and other newly developed cell culture techniques have promise, but they are expensive, unfinished—more hieroglyphics rather than less. Liver cancer has "successfully" been treated (higher rates of remission, smaller tumors) with radioactive antibodies specific to cancer cells. This is the best of both worlds, perhaps—a living drug that shines with deadly light inside, into the dark depths, rendering the person once again dangerous and radiant. But in a way, it works.

The wheat field must be weeded. Can it be justified to

give these drugs, these heavyweights, these hired killers, to a person in an early stage of cancer who may respond to a drug already tested? But how to refuse something that might work? What *are* we to do?

"**H**E WASN'T THERE AGAIN TODAY. I WISH, I WISH he'd stay away." That nagging ache in my left calf, that chronically swollen gland in my neck. I worry them like a child at a loose tooth, they worry me back. Some of us get cancer and others of us do not; what for me? In my own family, one has died of stomach cancer, one of cancer of the bone marrow, and one of a brain tumor. Another recently lost a breast, and more, from cancer. I slide my hands along my breasts with regularity, seeking, never sure what I would choose. Even quivering under the bedsheets I like to think of myself as a hardy specimen.

I recently read a scholarly article on hardiness. The author equated it with the ability to withstand pain, acclimate to new surroundings, thrive on change and stress. Perhaps I'm not so hardy after all. She proposed the notion that hardy people are in control of their lives when healthy and stay in control when sick—and specifically, they are more likely to survive cancer because of it. They don't *succumb*. Another queer kind of comfort for the ill, this unquantifiable characteristic. "The days wear on, but I endure," wrote Apollinaire, and we come full circle to the patient we all love to hate: the difficult one, the ones like Olive with the gall to remind us what the gaping holes in their bodies really hide. When she says of her wound, "This is my life," she is, in fact, embracing the tumor that has been cut away. I tell Richard about hardiness, but he already knows. "What if you had just six months to live?"

he asks me, reading a self-help book on managing your time. And he laughs when he says it.

WHAT A FINE JOKE ON ALL OF US IT WOULD BE WERE we to finally discover that cancer cured itself, or didn't—to find that all the drugs and surgeries were not the cure. There are, after all, so many miracle stories, so many coffee-table anecdotes of people who refused surgery on a tumor the size of a grapefruit and a month later it was gone. In these stories it is often the person who has turned his or her back on the treatment, embracing the tumor, who finds the redemptive cure.

We know so little. Cancer registries are less than thirty years old, such a tiny amount of time as to make conclusions about cancer in any historical sense meaningless. We have to learn to look at cancer in terms of major population shifts, longevity, changes in diet, climate, stress, and environment over centuries and millennia, not decades. We have to wonder what we will die of if we do cure cancer, what will take its place. Cancer has become a giant metaphor not just for hapless, worried people who finger their bodies and wonder; it is a symbol to many thousands of people who look at the world as a puzzle with its pieces all in disarray. If we cure cancer—never mind the subtle and not-so-subtle distinctions in "cure," in "cancer"—so much will be made clear. So many questions will be answered.

All this speculation, these ideas for me to turn in my hand like a shiny rock in the light: this is the easy part for me. I have nothing more immediate to grab my attention. I don't have a tumor gnawing at me, leaving its Cheshire grin long after the cat has gone.

PARAMETERS

I N MEDICINE, THERE IS AN ANSWER TO THE QUESTION "now what?" It is "all we can do." There is an answer to the question "How much?" It is "everything." By such a simple process as repetition, our whole expectation changes; what was once exotic is now routine. What is now exotic is rapidly becoming ordinary—even necessary. Medicine exists to keep the dying alive as long as possible, for we are all dying, we are all in failing health. Dialysis, cancer treatment: everyday stuff. Equal access for all.

This urge to classify, to name, to contain, requires a constantly shifting border: shifting outward. Whatever we have, we want more. In medicine a good part of the limit-pushing takes place in the intensive care units, where no one means to treat illnesses or effect a cure. Instead, it is a combination of stops pulled: it is meant to stave off, hold back, forestall. The intensive care unit (ICU) is painted with whispers, hushed thrills of concern from families, and the casual relaxation of the elite. It is a place to hang in the balance, to cling if you are the patient; it is a place to explore and create if you are the doctor. The barely alive make a bid at survival, often without asking, in beds beside the undiagnosed, the uncertain, the unable.

On television, intensive care seems to consist of secluded, private rooms, doors shut and no windows, no observers, where suspicious deaths and dramatic conversations can take place. Reality couldn't be more different. Intensive care wards are usually big rooms that hark back to Florence Nightingale's dormitories, with perhaps a few glassed-in desks that can be seen from the front desk. It is a designation of attitude as much as form, of supervision of the natural order as much as interference in it.

The walls behind the beds are banks of potential: suction, oxygen, monitors. Here a few small machines can sear the flesh intact—how fast, how rhythmically the heart beats, how the muscle moves, the valves flop open and snap closed. How is the blood pulsing through the body, how wide are the arteries, how fresh and free are the lungs. One has a semitransparent chest in ICU, and most of the questions are begun with the query "how." Data are gathered and examined, an accumulation of facts like an overnight snowfall. "We don't cure people here," says one of the nurses. "We just support their organs."

Mr. Lakey is here because he had a heart attack during open-heart surgery a few days ago. The surgery, a coronary bypass, was an attempt to open a channel of circulation to his malnourished heart muscle. That, at least, appears to be a success.

He is awake, drowsy but alert. Six bottles of intravenous fluid and medication flow into three different veins. He wears an opaque green mask, dewy with humidified oxygen. Urine drains from a catheter in his bladder. "It would be nice to sleep," says Mr. Lakey slowly, eminently weary. The mister makes a steady high whoosh in the tangle of tubes and poles that ties him in place and weaves through the armholes of his loose gown. Each bag of fluid costs $36, the tubing and needle $42, his bed another $800 each day.

Into Mr. Lakey's heart is threaded a long electrode. It floats in his pulmonary artery, the vessel feeding his lungs, and is held in place by a very small balloon. This balloon was inserted into a vein, rode the pulsing blood like a boat on a pounding surf, and sailed along through the upper chamber of his heart—then past the valves and through the lower chambers and out—down, down, down. This is a pulmonary pressure monitor, which measures in a fashion the efficiency of the heart's pumping. Such monitors are very common in critical care, part of the window on the chest that adds security to the clinical opinions of the physicians. It also adds a measure of risk to the patient, since the sliding ride of the balloon can excite and irritate the heart into dangerous, misbegotten rhythms.

Next to Mr. Lakey is a small black woman with big dark eyes, her mouth pursed and mute. She is apparently suffering from hepatic encephalopathy, a state of confusion and delirium brought on by poisons of the liver filling the bloodstream. It is often the end of long alcoholism, but this woman has no history of alcohol abuse. She is blank, flat, staring. A medical student talks to her, and she looks straight ahead or turns slowly to follow the pace of a person walking by. He keeps asking questions, embarrassed at her silence, a pleading tone rising in his voice.

In a bed beside her, not 8 feet away and unseparated by wall or curtain, is a woman in her midthirties. She is a dwarf, recovering from a surgery—not the first—aimed at correcting some of the curving, painful twists of her spine. To protect the cord and the incision, she is confined to a straight and rigid posture, on her side, propped by pillows. She is a small bump in the long, high bed, a mole.

In a room with walls of glass at the end of the ward lies Bill Potts. He is seventy-eight years old and looks ten years younger, a retired mountaineer who worked the high-altitude ranges of Europe. Yesterday his family was told that the pressure in his chest is a cancer that encircles the aorta, a tight bind around the major artery, pushing on his throat. Surgery cannot touch it, that delicate knot so near the heart. He began both chemotherapy and high-dose radiation yesterday, and it is vaguely hoped they will reduce the tumor to a more comfortable, hospitable size. Overnight his mind has begun to flicker and dim. His reflexes are odd, unpredictable. The tumor seems not to have noticed the x-rays, and it sits atop his chest in kingly glory. He breathes, for safety, on a ventilator, twenty-three breaths a minute, rapid and deep. Breathing in, breathing out.

The attending physician who supervises the medical residents strongly suggests at rounds that Mr. Potts would benefit from the same internal monitor that Mr. Lakey enjoys. "It would be interesting to document the diagnosis," he says. The resident is less than enthusiastic, never having inserted such a device alone, wondering about the restricted passage, the bulging tumor, the brittle heart, the point. When the attending physician is gone, one of the nurses jokingly suggests that the resident could effect a miracle cure. "We'll write a book," she tells him, "and get famous." He snorts. "There's two ways to find out what's going on—post and pre-post," he muses a few moments later. "We'll get the post anyway." He pauses. "But it *would* be interesting."

"**P**OST" AND "PRE-POST." ODD TERMS. A "POST" IS AN autopsy, a postmortem. "Pre-post," obviously, is before the autopsy—while the person lives. Other whimsical words abound here: a lung that wheezes or crackles with pneumonia has a "pulmonary imperfection"; the physical therapy given is a "pulmonary toilet." You die of "total body failure," or TBF.

In high-tech areas like ICU, "parameters" is a favorite word. Treatments and diagnostic tests are done to check parameters—boundaries—to set standards: in other words, to gather data. Once the standards are set and the proper routine designed, there is little backing out. Medicine is an ever-evolving escalation of technique, and in critical care more than any part of the hospital, one can see how the technique has made the inevitable unnatural, unthinkable.

People rarely have a simple death anywhere in a hospital; more often they "arrest," they are "coded," the last-ditch effort to revive the heart. Intensive care units set the rule, not the exception. Last night in this unit a ninety-four-year-old man in the last stages of heart disease and kidney failure had a heart attack (the most severe form, a cardiac arrest in which the heart completely stops) while he lay in the ICU unconscious. His regular physician, the doctor who had treated him through the course of his illness, was vacationing out of town. The doctor's associate who was left in charge refused to label the old man a "no-code," the appellation that would have prevented extraordinary life support measures. His reason was that the vacationing physician had already "lost" too many patients while he was out of town, and if there were any more, it would not be because his associate hadn't done anything to stop it.

When the man's heart stopped, a full resuscitation with drugs and electric shock was used to revive him. His heart began to beat again, and again, a few hours later, it stopped.

The code team revived him once more. He passed the night unconscious, and early this morning he had yet another cardiac arrest. After ten minutes of effort, the resident, chancing it, called off the team and the man died. The physician slept through the familiar ritual, the nurses' washing of the body and restocking of the code cart with medicine vials and syringes. The general opinion among the nurses and interns is that the resident did the right thing—but that little can be done to stop the same difficulty in the future.

ONE MAN I REMEMBER IN PARTICULAR; ALTHOUGH I bathed him and gave him medicine and brushed his teeth and talked with his wife, I never saw him alive. He was dead all the days I cared for him. I was in the last weeks of nursing school and assigned to shadow an experienced nurse in the ICU. I learned how to read monitors and heart rhythm strips and the way a cardiologist walks. Midway through my tour I was assigned to help care for a man, a forty-five-year-old man visiting his children from his home 1000 miles away. He had stood up from dinner with a pain in his chest, walked into the hospital's emergency room a few hours later, and dropped to the floor without a heartbeat. The code team restored it and took him unconscious to ICU.

In the next five days he had seventeen more cardiac arrests. Each time he was brought back to a kind of life. Each arrest sent little shock waves through his brain, and its herringbone trellis grew dark and bruised with tiny strokes. On the second day, an EEG revealed only vague, lost waves, wandering sighs. On the third day an x-ray sliced up a picture of his brain like a breadloaf and showed a herniation. The brain itself had shifted, was being sucked down into the top of the spinal column by the growing pressure of blood in his skull. By then his heart would not keep beating for more than a few moments without the amphetamine that dripped through his IV.

One is inclined to wonder what the point might be. My hands knew he was dead; it was a message that skin could tell skin. It was a message his eyes could tell anyone who gazed in them with an open heart and not just a penlight. A body flaccid and warm, sallow and soft, unmoving, uncaring, unsparked—but breathing in the queer regularity of the ventilated. Breathing in, breathing out.

What was the point? The nurses were told, obliquely, in the evasive manner of medicine, that it was for his wife's sake. It was so she could have time to absorb the difficult knowledge that her husband would die, and die young. I think of him and I think of Aaron, and how the natural becomes abnormal, the obvious obscure. What kind of death is harder to bear witness to—the unexpected and sudden or the slow and delayed? What is worse—to permit the inevitable or be forced to choose it? After five days, his wife had to sign the papers allowing the doctors to turn off the drugs, unplug the machines.

I T IS OBVIOUS TO THE NURSES AND RESIDENTS THAT BILL Potts won't improve. ICU was a stepping-stone until his prognosis was clear—a step either to the medical wards or the morgue. He came to have his parameters defined, his data gathered.

When the day shift is 2 hours old, Bill Potts's monitor beeps a calm warning, that he is having an episode of ventricular tachycardia—"v-tach"—when the lower chambers of the heart beat very rapidly and overwhelm the regular beat normally controlled by a node in the upper chambers. "Don't worry, he's a no-code," one nurse says to another when the alarm sounds.

Miracle monitors, these screens at the bedside and the nurses' desk. One can perch on a stool in front of a row of screens, each screen with three moving lines, each line corresponding to a patient. With a flip of a switch, a printed readout of the heart rhythm rolls from a nearby slit. With a push of a button, a screen changes to a graphic display of one person's pulse, respiration, blood pressure, and pulmonary artery pressure. The large white room is reduced to thin green tracings by the monitors, all the room in a glance from one seat.

The moment of ventricular tachycardia was Bill Potts's valediction. His heart jitterbugged and then waltzed, slowing to a two-step and then beating a beguine. A "normal" pulse would range from 60 to 90 beats a minute; within a half-hour his heart rate has slowed to 30-odd irryhthmic beats a minute, in what is ironically called an "agonal rhythm." These wave swells are erratic and of little help to a body now starved for oxygen. One by one the nurses, residents, and interns move from his bed to the desk 10 yards away, gathering round the monitors, eating handfuls of almonds from a can on a nearby shelf. Every few minutes someone reaches over and flips the switch for a printout. The alarms are turned off now because they would beep without stop for this unnatural pattern. Translated to paper and ink, this pattern is called the "dying heart."

Bill Potts's eyes are half-open, and with each controlled breath his chest jumps slowly and his head bounces lightly backward, almost in slow motion. His room is empty of people; his heart has slowed to fifteen tired spasms a minute. The respiratory technician climbs off the high stool by the desk at 10:04 a.m. and walks to his bedside to turn off the ventilator. Bill Potts's breathing stops; the irregular curviforms flatten out. At 10:08 a.m. the resident calls death, casually, to the nurse sitting beside him. She scribbles a quick note. Even then the flat line bounces now and again, hill and dale every several seconds. The electrical fibers of the heart shoot and quiver and bristle—they will for days—like the leg of a dreaming dog.

Another resident, a lithe, dark woman, walks to the bedside to disconnect the IV and monitor. She reaches over to slide Potts's eyes closed, but they open again. "It's not like in the movies," she laughs, a bit embarrassed by his stare, "when they stay closed."

T OM SPENCE WORKED EIGHT YEARS IN THE ARMY MEDICAL corps; then he went to college for a degree in nursing. He has been in critical care for several years and is a member of the committee that makes policy on life support and codes. He is brash, confident, overfrank, a tall, clean-cut man with strong opinions and a self-conscious manner that holds others slightly at bay. What he sees as the feminine passivity of nursing grates on Tom. "The nurse-doctor relationship, the struggle to get credit for what I can do, is the real source of stress here," he says. He feels that the interns and residents take the praise for his good ideas and blame him if his ideas don't work: "They'll turn around and say, 'It was the *nurse's* idea,' " he grimaces.

Medical students, interns, and residents all come and go on the unit in rapid succession, often spending only six weeks here before moving to an entirely different part of the hospital. The nurses are here day after day, and most consider themselves specialists. Some have postgraduate certification in critical care and advanced life support. Taking orders from new faces can make them chafe a bit roughly under the bit. It is one of the paradoxical trials of the nurse that she or he must learn a fair amount of medical theory to survive. For example, before giving a medicine a nurse is legally responsible for ascertaining that the physician has ordered a correct dose, at correct times, and in the proper fashion. A nurse who follows an incorrect medical order can be sued for negligence. (Nurses can be sued for malpractice, too, but it is less than clear cut. Malpractice is a crime only a professional can commit; some judges have declared that nursing did not fit the criteria for a profession. In such an instance a nurse is sued for negligence, and her conduct is compared, according to the law, only to the conduct of "an ordinary prudent person," regardless of whether an ordinary person would ever have the skills relevant to the claim of negligence—like starting arterial lines, injecting epinephrine, managing a dialysis machine, or transfusing blood. In some cases a nurse's conduct has been judged according to a physician's opinion of how she or he should have behaved.)

Because the orders go only one way—down—physicians never need learn anything of nursing philosophy and skill. A surprising number of doctors, including young doctors, scoff at the idea that nurses consider their job to be a separate discipline, a profession. The controversy of who gets credit can be most acute in the technical specialties, where the physicians make choices of life and death, but the nurse must carry them out.

Surgeons, especially, lack respect for the nurses in the ICU unit, says Tom. Midway through the afternoon, long after Bill Potts's body has been wheeled away to the morgue, an attractive and carefully dressed young woman enters the unit. She approaches two scrub-clad men with stethoscopes around their necks and beepers on their belts. One leans on the nurses' desk, the other sits at the computer terminal, feet jutting out into the aisle. "I'm looking for someone on the medical staff," she smiles at them. "You two look like medical types." The doctor seated at the computer swallows the mouthful of almonds he's been thoughtfully chewing. "We're not medical types," he grins, speaking sharply. "We're surgeons! And we're busy." The woman's smile turns cool as the tall, gangly surgeon stands up, towering over her, to point at the medical resident down the room. "Now that you've stood up," she says in a slow voice, derisive, looking him up and down, "I can see that." The surgeon misses her sarcasm and reaches for another handful of nuts as he watches her walk away.

T OM RETURNS FROM LUNCH TO FIND MR. LAKEY'S TUBES trundled up, a stretcher by his bed, ready for a trip to the radiation lab below. Although there are no symptoms of the condition, a physician suspects Mr. Lakey of having a pulmonary embolus, a blockage of part of the blood circulation to the lung usually caused by a clot. He plans to do a V-Q study, which measures the ventilation-perfusion ratio of the lung and can identify areas of blockage. Tom argues with the physician, the orderly who is to help with the transfer, the head nurse. He is offended and repeats the morning's findings to the doctor, that Tom had checked for signs of a pulmonary embolus and found no evidence of one. Tom's nursing judgment and examination skills are at stake, he feels. He loses the argument.

Moving a patient with multiple intravenous lines, monitors, oxygen, and a pulmonary pressure line is not simple or safe. Tom, the orderly, and the physician all accompany Mr. Lakey on his journey down a narrow elevator to the lab two floors below and along a long, bumpy hallway in the old wing of the hospital to have his V-Q study done.

In a room crowded with bulbous machines larger than the people standing between them, the sedated Mr. Lakey is prepared for the test, which costs about $400. His stretcher is slid between the projecting arms of a machine that reads radioactivity and projects the resulting "picture" on a screen, taking still photographs in the process. Drowsy, he breathes a mist filled with a suspended low-radiation isotope, and immediately the screen fills with a pointillist silhouette of the lungs, the dots filling in the picture from the center out as the mist is spread through the lung tissue. Several minutes pass as photos are taken of each aspect of both lungs. Then a liquid isotope is injected into one of Mr. Lakey's IV lines and moves within seconds through the heart to the pulmonary circulation. Again, the screen fills with a lung shape in white on black. The pictures of air movement and blood flow are almost identical, showing none of the blocked areas characteristic of an embolus. Tom is vindicated.

Part of the baggage that accompanied the entourage to the lab was a portable Life-Pak monitor and defibrillator. This machine provides the same continuous track of the heartbeat as the permanent screens in the intensive care unit and has attached to it the electric paddles that can be used to stimulate a stopped heart. It rolls along beside the stretcher, leashed to Mr. Lakey's chest by electrode wires. In the lab, the monitor line suddenly failed, the screen went blank. Tom and the physician were left without a heart rhythm to watch. After Mr. Lakey is safely returned to his room, Tom sets out to investigate the problem and discovers that the batteries are dead.

A few months later, two defibrillator manufacturers issued a recall for over 11,000 machines like the Life-Pak. The batteries showed "an abnormally high self-discharge rate," said a spokesman.

How very different doctors and nurses are. this difference and the conflicts it inevitably creates are much of my job. We, nurses, talk about them, doctors, all through a work day, in short phrases, rolled eyes, and one-word epithets. The relationship is not one of smooth team-work, even when individuals move against the general stream. The difference is fundamental, a difference in purpose and motive. This is part of the point, this comple-mentarity, a tesselation of skill and concern. By discipline, we are interested in different aspects of the same thing—the patient. At times the distinction seems a great, echoing gulf across which I yell in vain—for they can't hear me. Are they listening? Do they call to me when my back is turned, my attention distracted? Am I calling in the right words, in the right language?

A few weeks ago I came to work early in the morning to discover that one of my patients—who happened to be a physician who'd suffered some brain damage—had an in-filtrated intravenous line. The needle and tubing meant to drip fluid into his vein had slipped through its thin wall, dripping into the muscle and fat tissue of his arm. The arm and hand were swollen, cold and hard. I took the needle out, we argued over whether I would bring him an ice pack or a warm soak. "I'm the doctor," he told me with gritted teeth, and so he was. He demanded the ice. I gave him what he wanted.

I'm not very good at starting IVs. Give me a young fellow and that big vein in the hollow of the elbow and I can get blood almost every time in one stick. But I haven't that fine, intuitive touch for slipping a small, short needle in a slippery little vein on the back of the hand, doing it by feel, by art. When possible, I defer to the specialists, the nurses who spend their working days carrying a basket of needles and bandages from room to room.

The IV therapy nurse came to my patient's bed and poked here, patted there, while he goaded and protested, with a sour, sarcastic smile. She was unsuccessful and left to call her colleague. In the meantime, the man's own physician and her two residents, heeling like pets, arrived for rounds. When I explained that the IV therapist had thus far been unable to begin the IV, she was unhappy. I was berated. "If *I* have to come off my rounds to start this IV, I'm going to be angry," she told me, as though I wanted to know, as though I cared. She assumed I would listen. "It's ridiculous—he's got good veins." She turned briefly to the patient who watched with the same smile and glittering eyes; he was, after all, a doctor. "I just don't understand this," she said at last and strode away, pushing the door as she left so that it banged against the closet behind it.

Most doctors fancy themselves experts at starting IVs, and indeed most of them are. But it is not because of a greater artistic talent—it is because of the singlemindedness that cuddles up to the heart of medicine.

IVs hurt; everyone knows that. One reason I'm not good at them is my lack of nerve, the way I back down when the patient pulls away or complains. In a sense, this is a failure on my part, a cowardice. It is precisely why a doctor will succeed where I can't: pain—others' pain—doesn't slow their progress or dog their steps. Once the decision to slide a needle between skin cells is made, it will be done. (My friend Richard, the physician's assistant, also works parttime in a hospital, drawing blood samples early in the morning. Sometimes he can't bring himself to wake a slumbering patient with the needle, and leaves it to the physician to take the blood later. But Richard says his softheartedness probably backfires: whenever this happens he comes to work the next day to find the patients' arm bruised and swollen from the doctor's efforts. "Their veins are ruined," he says. "It happens every time.") A doctor will tighten that tourniquet and slap those vessels and poke and prick and poke some more until the fluid flows. The will be done. Like the resident holding the sick baby, he won't coo, he won't sing or dream. He won't even look up.

T HE THIRD ADMISSION OF THE SHIFT IS ARRIVING IN MID-afternoon. He is a coronary artery bypass graft— CABG—patient, a triple, who recently had a severe heart attack. Bypass patients are known as cabbages, for CABG. You say "the cabbage in room 205," and of course you mean the man who had the bypass. But I always see a great vegetable, pale and wan, overflowing the sheets.

He rolls in, accompanied by several nurses and physicians in scrub suits, with nine IV bags hanging above the stretcher, one filled with blood to replace what he lost in the operation. The physicians drift to the walls and the desk, leaning back and watching as the nurses pounce on the patient like ants on a dead beetle, rapidly and systematically passing bags and tubing from the portable poles to the permanent ones by the bedside, hooking him from the portable monitors to the permanent monitors. Conversation fills the room and spills into the ward. "Which one is the pacer line?" "What's the baseline BP?" A surgeon perches on the empty stretcher, back to the wall, feet sticking out in front of him, and watches the numbers on the green monitor change. Tubes stitched into the man's freshly closed chest bubble a froth of blood into a large plastic jar on the floor beside the bed, where a nurse crouches to read the measurement.

His blood pressure is dropping, disconcertingly. His heart is erratic, potassium levels low. Another argument ensues: How much IV potassium? How fast? until a clear order from one of the physicians is called out louder than the others and no one contradicts it.

He won't die here, not after all this, not after this effort and teamwork and all this money. But he might code at any time—and may we all have mercy on his soul.

ENOUGH. HEART-BEATING CADAVERS, AFTER ALL, BE-come just cadavers in time. I am ready to leave, I seek the door that leads away. I wander to the morgue, and it is a long way away, down abandoned flights of stairs that echo my steps, where the handrail is covered with dust. The business upstairs fades with the distance the way a dream fades, growing fainter and more transparent, till the details and point are forgotten.

The tables are high, cold, white steel, shaped like troughs. The body of a man lies atop one, several hours dead, stiffening but still full of warmth. He is elderly, fat, bald but for a wild fringe of gray hair circling his scalp. He has two days' growth of beard, no teeth, and his jaw hangs askew. His eyes are open, chalk blue. He gazes benignly at the ceiling. He is naked. One leg has been cut off at the mid-thigh and the stump looks ragged and torn.

Two pathologist's assistants will work on this case. They are called "dieners," from a German word for "valet." I want my hands in too, to get the blood on them.

The first cut is a Y across the chest, with the three points aimed at the armpits and the belly. The pale skin folds back in a sigh, and Steve, one of the dieners, works at the yellow fat. When he reaches the muscle, the blood begins to run and doesn't stop; it pools ceaselessly in the cavities and drains down the sloping table to the pipes at the lowest end. He pulls the muscles away from the bone, roughly, and picks up a small circular saw.

Ten years ago I stepped into my human anatomy and physiology class as though it were the shores of the New World and plunged my hands into the cadavers without hesitation. I took pride in the fact that I wasn't squeamish, that I was content to dissect alone in the laboratory. What eager student has room for irresolution?

Times have changed. These bodies are different; they bleed, their warmth seeps through my gloves as I reach under a stomach, around a loop of intestine. And I know them; I've washed these faces, held these hands.

The blade bites through the ribs with quick, whining slices, bumping along the uneven surface. In a few moments the entire ribcage is lifted clear of the man, like the breastplate off a suit of armor. The viscera are exposed, a rainbow of enamel paint, a bowl of shiny, slippery secrets.

"Big heart," says the knife-wielder, hefting the tough, fat-covered organ. He cuts through the translucent membranes that hold the chest in place, and then everything comes out in one quilted pile, to be dropped in a large steel basin between the man's thighs: heart, lungs, aorta, a lumpy, mottled liver, everything. The bladder slides out, with a catheter still attached. The other diener, a small Asian woman, reaches under the pelvic bone and pulls out the testicles.

The body slides on the table, the hands bouncing with each jar. The man wears a plain gold band on the left ring finger. I can see nothing but blood in the tureen left of the man's belly. He is like a big soup cauldron, simmering broth. Steve pulls his wet gloves out and gives them a shake, moving away from the intestines he's been poking at and turning to the top of the table, to the head.

We are in a teaching hospital today. One never forgets the constant need for specimens. The pile of organs between his legs will go to the weekly organ conference and then be burned. His brain, says Steve, will go to "brain-cutting conference." Here, at least, words mean what they say.

He props the man's head on a block, as though the fellow were trying to peer at his feet. The first cut, an incision in the back of the head, is made with a butcher knife. As the membrane holding the scalp is sliced, Steve rolls the skin forward, ear to ear. Within a few minutes he has wound up the scalp like the top of a Spam can and gives one final tug over the man's eyes. He is blindfolded by his skin. The uncombed hair, bloody now, tickles his chin.

"Stand back a bit," Steve warns me. "This smells like the dentist." The circular saw cuts through the skullcap. Bits of blood and brain fly. Then he picks up a shiny steel wedge and pries at the bone, in a small triangular nick he'd prepared. "Like cutting a jack-o'-lantern, so the top doesn't fall in when you put it back on." Crack, crack. In a moment the bowl pops off into his hand and he lays it aside.

Little holds the brain in place: its stem, the animal brain, narrows to the cord as it disappears down a long tunnel of vertebrae. Here it parts with little protest. From the eye sockets lead the two optic nerves, a few millimeters wide and creamy white. Much smaller, almost threads, the many other cranial nerves hang loosely.

I am holding the brain in my hands. It is warm, soft, spongy, slippery. I see where the saw has bitten into the tissue, one vertical slice across the convoluted indentations.

I N THE SPECIMEN ROOM NEXT DOOR ARE JARS. TONGUES, eyes, a whole foot, an ovary as big as a cantaloupe. Who are all these people? How many have I bathed, stroked, spoken to, spoken about? What are they doing upstairs anyway? What *is* going on? Where have they taken Bill Potts and his wondrous tumor?

Crackerjack boxes are nothing to these buckets, these surprises. I open a plastic tub of brains, another of bowel. I see a box of dried cobwebs, unidentifiable in the dim light. At eye level is a gallon container, white, filled with fluid and something heavy and tightly bound in that small space.

The lid is tight; this jar has not been opened for a long while. I have to hold it up against my chest to tug at the top, but finally, the afternoon almost gone, the room quiet, suspended, I open the jar. I open it and find a newborn baby.

A voice drifts through the door from the bright room where the blood runs. With a sudden chill I recognize her. I recognize them all. These are the remnants of our good intentions, of our failures, of all the well-meaning heads bent low over a lab table, over a microscope, over a needle and syringe. And high above me, far away, I can still hear the quiet hum of machines, breathing in, breathing out.

VOODOO

O N MY DESK, WITHIN ARM'S REACH, IS A COMMON BOOK
called *Taber's Cyclopedic Medical Dictionary*. I skim *Taber's* now and then, either to read a succinct summary of
a particular condition or state (habenular trigone, or par-
amnesia, or tetanus antitoxin) or to check the spelling of
a word. In the back of this elegant and understated book,
with its green fake-leather cover and engraved gold let-
tering, are tables: metric equivalents, commonly accepted
laboratory values, drug interactions, and such. The other
day I was flipping through it, looking for nothing in particular, when I suddenly noticed a table I'd never seen
before: "Miracles of the Body," it said, and was gone, the
pages flipping too fast for me to catch. I was awake then,
paying attention. Miracles? In *Taber's*? Is this a secret I've
missed, a chapter I should have read a long time ago? I
almost felt betrayed, for a brief, unthinking second. Is

this a new specialty, some subset of medicine I'd never known? So back I went, flipping the pages, trying to catch it, and there it was. "Muscles of the Body," it said. "Muscles." I'd not missed anything after all.

There are no miracles in medicine, and precious little reverence. No thanks are given for opportunities, no time spent discussing the boundaries of behavior, of proper attitude, of the possibility that something is sacred. This lack of veneration, of honor given, has in recent years become impious. I don't think, though, that it is the mocking, sad disrespect of a disillusioned adult, shaking his fist at a God he feels betrayed by. Not at all. The irreverence I see practiced so casually around the sick is the irreverence of small children witnessing a cataclysm. It is just more whistling in the dark. So small, so inadequate, so lacking in understanding, we rush pell-mell, head down and eyes closed, to prove ourselves.

Little boys get silly when they're bored. And they get silly when a sudden clap of thunder shakes the house, when someone jumps out at them from behind a door, when on Halloween night a skeleton hangs from the ceiling. Medicine is silly in just this way. Faced with overwhelming complexity, with subtlety beyond comprehension, medicine has trained itself to see only black and white. All this happens below consciousness, and it is flavored by the fear at its heart. Why do physicians walk away from the bedside before the respirator stops? Why do they speak of diseases and not the diseased?

This is the scientific method of living one's life. It works for solving certain problems—therefore, it will work for a world view. It is the Midas touch of medicine, that the sick and suffering are forgotten so that their illnesses can be healed. Pigeons are squeezed into their requisite holes. Such a life as I—and others—have the chance to live, spending my days at the beds of people dying—such a life should broaden the mind and heart in ways little else can do, like certain paintings, measures of music, poem fragments. This is direct experience, free of theory. Why do we become inured to it, bored, seeking a greater distance? Why do we push it away, turn our backs? For we'll only seek it elsewhere, not knowing its name. Do we expect too much of ourselves—am I asking too much of myself, of others, that every day we should change a little, learn?

I know how it works, I can follow the biochemistry well enough. I know that B follows A, the methodology, the equations that solve for x. I am, in truth, fascinated by the forms and language of science. This is the key to the pleasure. This is why I read *Taber's* for fun. What an impossible and rare animal the human being is. For this reason alone, I can understand the preoccupation. What can be seen can often be described by a series of cell divisions and chemical reactions laid end to end, a puzzle to be solved. But so much cannot be seen. We are like the nineteenth-century physicists who thought, before Einstein's rude awakening, it was possible to know the answers, all of them. Damn the meaning; we're here to catalog.

The greatest puzzle medicine faces, the jigsaw with pieces missing, is that so much can't be seen. What happens to black and white then? The endless classification of symptom and disease will never be an explanation, no kind of explanation at all for the experience of being sick, for the effect sickness has on a person, on the people who care for that person. For medicine to heal, it must make sense of what cannot be seen and revere it. We need a morality of the evanescent and inexplicable; from there we might approach a moral treatment of health and illness.

ONE MORALITY TALE REMAINS TO BE TOLD; I SAVE IT for last because it is in many ways an extended metaphor and because it is about a particular blindness. This is the fable of animals and how they serve us in our cause. "Living animals are the proving grounds of ideas that cannot be tested on people," says a scientist, and already he's speaking in tongues. People, animals—two separate classes. And both in cages. Research animals are the cement that binds together the disparate should-have-dieds and the dubious gifts given to them in their extra hours. We treat them like sick people, only more so. Animals are bodies, perfect bodies, without a soul or a complaint. They are mechanisms, and their use is a specialty as precise as neurosurgery—and as elite.

This specialty has its own language, a dialect not unlike the dialects of cancer and critical care. These equivocal and double-tongued words serve many purposes. They distance the researchers from nonresearchers, from the work, intimidate outsiders. The distance and abbreviation increase the camaraderie of the specialists and create a sense of membership—a membership that is strengthened by the threats and criticism of outsiders. Creating new words where old ones would suffice, putting old words to new uses is a way to claim extraordinary worth for the work. The project in question and those in charge are elevated to a point where mere English, the language of everyday use, is inadequate to describe it. It goes beyond routine matters.

Most significantly, the language of research boxes in the animals themselves, defining them and categorizing them, until they are comfortably placed below and far away. This is the essential way animals are like sick people: they are different. It is assumed they appreciate our efforts.

In this world, starvation becomes deprivation; pain and loud noises become aversive stimuli and negative reinforcement; killing becomes sacrifice. (Almost ironic, the use of the word "sacrifice" here, with its religious overtones. One thinks of the baboon killed so its heart could be transplanted into Baby Fae—that animal was called a "donor.") The animals become first organisms, then models, and finally, resources. Then we can talk about resource conservation. If the organism withdraws from pain, it is demonstrating a reaction to sensation. If it screams or cries out when subjected to negative reinforcement, it is said to vocalize. If it keeps screaming, it vocalizes continuously.

Here is an elitism so complete, so self-sufficient, that it encloses an entire view of the world and one's place in it. The language provides an abbreviated method for closing off all meaning that fails to meet one's needs, that is uncomfortable or difficult or irritating. You can get a lot done without lingering over niceties. All is neatly subdivided. Each member has a role. This is the true heart of the language and the distance. In order to justify using them as machines, as instruments of science, monkeys "react to sensations" rather than "feel pain," and their reactions are seen as scientific data. Not to worry that a monkey's reaction is any more or less objective than a burn patient's pain. A system for describing both will be found.

Every day has an agenda. The sick *will* be cured. The blind will see; the lame will walk again—in a fashion. Certainly the sick will be subjected to a great deal of inspection and a number of sincere attempts to influence and redirect. They are caged first by ill health and then by their treatment. The sick are caged like animals, and in the same way that we justify what we do to sick people for the hoped-for end—a miracle before breakfast and what is left to discuss?—so animals are treated as they are for the possible rewards.

I must note that researchers are quick to point out, and

have pointed out to me a number of times, that animals also benefit from animal research. This seems a bit like saying that an organ donor benefits by his or her donation. A successful surgery and a dead patient still leave you with a successful surgery, after all. As for animals: new ways to combat infection and improved veterinary techniques do derive from research. The occasional animal may benefit. Most interesting, though, is that I am told that the animal in the lab *lives longer* than its companions in the wild. So does the human being on the ventilator. In the wild the predator snatches its prey, and life is a series of narrow escapes and close calls. In the laboratory, as in the medical wards—well, it all depends on the day's agenda. The consequences of aggression, of the need to know, are great. Allow me to describe a few.

We have bullet-wound laboratories and radiation laboratories, studies on head injuries that involve slamming monkeys and dogs into walls, similar studies to develop better helmet protection for boxers and football players. We have animals pinned in metal chairs for months, to learn about immobility. There is an entire journal called *Pain*.

The call is out for more "animal models of chronic pain." Many researchers have written that animals do not feel, at least not in the same way that humans do. Their pain is mild, perhaps, or unremembered, or unimportant. Perhaps, like burn and cancer patients, half the pain they claim is mere anxiety.

A peculiar example of the kind of thinking involved here is the following statement by Dr. Orville Smith. At the time he was director of a federally funded primate research center in Washington. He is talking about the restraint chair, a device in which an animal is tied, by means of metal, leather, or cloth bands, for a period of time—some monkeys stay in restraint chairs for as long as a year. The restraint is used most often in pain studies.

Dr. Smith says his researchers dislike using it and so developed an alternative method, a cage that can turn into a temporary chair. "When it's time to run tests, the animal hops onto the seat and sticks his head through the top of the cage. We give him a little piece of apple and wheel the whole cage into the study room. When the testing is done, the seat is removed and the animal is back in his cage."

Now, I don't know exactly what kind of tests Dr. Smith is running on these animals, but I wonder at the idea of spirited volunteerism his statement conveys. The restraint chair was developed to spare the researchers frequent struggles and the tedious task of tying knots and fastening handcuffs. How cooperative will most animals be, apple or no—how cooperative slaves, inmates, prisoners—in saving their masters that precious time? What kind of blinders must be worn in order to see the test animal as a kind of dumb but willing accomplice in the whole thing?

Pain recently published an article that illustrates nicely the point of all this. The author hoped to prove, in part, that morphine relieved chronic pain. Never mind that there already exists a rather large body of literature on the subject. There is always more to learn.

The authors mention two problems with pain research—"aside from ethical considerations." The first is the difficulty in producing pain that is "persistent" over a long time. The second is "validation"—how to know that the animal really feels pain and how much pain it is feeling. Many studies use vocalization to test this, summoning up various methods for testing the "vocalization threshold." But the need for validation led these scientists to study a peculiar behavior called "autotomy."

"Autotomy" means self-cutting; it is mutilation by an animal of a part of its body. Investigators have developed an autotomy scale to objectively describe its intensity: the scale begins with (for paws) the tips of one or more nails removed, then steps up to one or more nails removed and damage to the ends of the digits, and ends with one or more digits removed. Each step is worth a certain number of points. The point value is added up for a total autotomy score.

In this study, pain was induced in two ways. First, on a hot plate, heated to approximately 135 degrees Fahrenheit, on which the rats were placed until they began licking their hind paws or until forty seconds had elapsed, whichever came first. Second, their tails were shocked with electricity until vocalization, and this was repeated until each individual animal's vocalization threshold was established.

One group of rats, under anesthesia, was implanted with pumps that delivered a continuous amount of either morphine or naltrexone, a chemical that blocks morphine and similar substances, including the natural opiates made by the body. ("Rats showing neurological deficits postoperatively were discarded," we are informed.) Then, using hot plate and shock, the researchers compared the "latency to licking the paw," compared the vocalization threshold to the first attempts. They must have been busy for days, weeks, bent over their desks and tabletops. A new piece—well, not new exactly, as everyone knows, but similar, a validation, a replication, a holding of the known up to the light in order to say, yes, this is what it was before, it is the same—was added to the puzzle. Morphine reduces pain. And aren't we glad to know?

Here's another, just briefly: "A typical experiment protocol involves rats exposed to escapable shock and yoked controls to inescapable shock. In several studies, accelerated tumor growth occurred for animals exposed to inescapable, uncontrollable stress." If this is surprising, and perhaps it is not, what have we learned? Well, admits the writer, not much. "Application of this research to humans, however, may be difficult." Thus is the obvious made objective, common sense turned into scientific truth, the apparent made manifest. It is not enough that we assume through our own rich experience of the world that certain things are true, that certain likelihoods can be expected. Each must be proved, proved many times, each proof subjected to exhausting repetition to determine its accuracy.

Not all the suffering is for the sake of pain. A group of researchers studying tastebud development wondered at the capacity of the fetus to taste what it swallows. They put pregnant ewes under anesthesia and cut open their uteruses. In some experiments the still-living fetuses were exposed to certain "taste stimuli" and then, still on the table, their brains were dissected so that changes in the cells could be observed. In another experiment, the fetal sheep—shockingly, born for just a few moments—were fitted with tubes that ran into their noses, mouths, and in some cases, brains. Thus outfitted, they were plunged back into the wombs and tied in place, the tube running out the mother's skin. At their leisure, for weeks, the researchers squirted bits of sugar and salt, snacks of bitter and sour and acid, down the tube, wondering at the baby's response.

What could possibly be the meaning of all this punishment? The researchers, asked such a question, look up blankly for a moment, and then return to the microscope. The meaning, of course, is obvious. It is medicine on the move, research at its best, its most inspired. A cure will be found, suffering somehow ended. These are the limits of biochemistry and mechanism. There can't be any greater meaning than what is seen.

I N THE LAST FEW YEARS, ANIMAL RESEARCHERS HAVE BEEN under fire, called to justify their work and its results.

Lots of talk goes by about the "ethics" of it, talk that seems to grow more arcane by the day. If four people and a dog are in a lifeboat, who can be thrown overboard if the boat is sinking? Is it "wrong" to choose the dog or "right"? What if it weighs less than the humans? What if one of the humans owns the boat? Do children matter more? Yes, but what if the dog is very famous and a rare, expensive breed? What then?

Whole books are devoted to "proving" whether or not animals are inferior to humans, and whether or not humans have the "right" to use them for human gain. Or if humans and animals are in the same spectrum. Much of the talk centers on our "capacity for enrichment," expressed—and therefore, thank heaven, quantifiable—in the amount of products external to ourselves that we produce, in our appreciation of what we are capable of doing.

We produce art, music, and books full of ideas, each idea derived in a sequential fashion; we construct buildings, bridges, and oil derricks; we blast tunnels and manufacture soap and tissue paper. We act on the world; we make our own existence manifest and force the world to change. We also act on each other. Animals—well, they just go about their business, building nests and such, flying around the clouds and singing, eating each other, and making babies. So there you have it.

All this building and tearing down, all our painting and symphony composing—this is our capacity to live rich lives. But skim away the poetry and you see that the real proof of our superiority over animals is our ability to use them—that is, we have the right to use them because we *can*, because *we* built the labs and hot plates and electroshock machines, *we* write the anatomy books, *we* apply for the grants.

We do experiment on humans, as even the most shallow reading of medicine must demonstrate. But we muck it all up, call it something else, a study or an investigation. We bury it in consent forms and interviews, permission slips, documentation, and good intentions. Why do we bother? Any person lying on his or her back, staring at the ceiling while the needle slides in, cares not a whit for a permission slip. Burned Nancy, urine-soaked Molly— they just want out. That old, dying woman, drinking the new cancer drug into her veins, dreaming of a miracle, a fantastic kind of parole—what matters the words? The sick are all just rats yoked up to inescapable, uncontrollable shocks. Untie them, and most of them just sit there, not knowing where a door might be.

"I HAVE TO LOOK AT YOUR SKIN," I TELL AN ELDERLY woman, newly come to our care. There is no delicate way to put this; I want to see her naked, see the telltale redness that warns of a coming bedsore, see the friction burns and heat rashes and bruises that the chronically ill carry like battle scars. She is an irritable, often angry woman. She is ninety-three years old, uses oxygen to walk across her room, and takes an hour to dress in a nightgown and robe. I don't know how she will respond to my impertinent request.

Hefting breathlessly to her feet, she drops her robe to the floor and lifts her shimmering blue gown up to her neck; she stands there impassive, silent, while I inspect her. She has a "dowager's hump," a mass like Quasimodo's rising between her shoulders, pressing her head toward her chest. She is shaped like a small, ornamental tree; her legs are the thin, straight trunk, her round back, pendulous belly and flat breasts the spherical crown. Her skin is extraordinarily dry and hangs in layers off her arms and back. I lift first one breast, then the other, peer under her arms, between her legs. Nothing escapes my attention. What a fine adjustment to the sick role this difficult patient has made! She knows there is no escape. She knows she is yoked for life.

The greater the similarity to humans, the greater the value of the animal in the experiment—so the money is more useful and the results of monkey experiments more meaningful than those on mice or rabbits or cats. But turn the tables and the animal suddenly becomes foreign, dissimilar, alien. One of the squirrel monkeys taken on the space shuttle in April of 1985 bit a trainer's finger and chewed on a stethoscope as he was being caged. "They are vicious, and there is nothing lovable about them," said the mission commander, apparently surprised at the animal's ungrateful reaction. None of these monkeys were given names—as space monkeys have had in the past—because the scientists didn't want to "humanize" them. This convenient fluidity in the nature of the animal—or patient—is not for their benefit, indeed. It is for ours.

Any product, any chemical, any surgical procedure finds its way to the human level sooner or later, and the first trial on humans is the only one that counts. Human trials are always essentially blind, because we're *not* monkeys. From monkeys we can perfect techniques, twists of the wrist, but we can't learn the truth of human health and disease. For that we need humans.

And we have them: a group of men half-jokingly referred to by a surgeon as the "World Series" of the artificial heart. It seems he meant that one doesn't give up on the series if the first few games are lost. We have Baby Faes and Baby Doe (and Doe and Doe). And we have all the other animals.

The animal researchers, fretful, tell me there is no bridge, no way to cross this gulf. I am one of those "misguided" people, sentimental, illogical. One researcher grants patronizingly that people opposed to animal research mean well but don't "understand science." They—we—are "animal lovers," extremists who would have us throw out the baby with the bathwater, the hot plate with the rat.

We parcel out pain, a bit here, a lot there. How can we even begin to talk about medical ethics in this position? To balance degrees of grief is to walk a knife-edge, sure to slip. It can't be done. This is the temptation of the Grand Inquisitor—lay your freedom at his feet. All humanity to be happy forever, but standing on one weeping, tortured child. All humanity. Can you walk away from such temptation?

Ah, but they are just animals after all. Who can say they aren't glad to lay their lives down for us, to ease our suffering some small bit? Our praises are sung by birds and beasts alike; they sing of our skill in a chorus of continuous vocalization.

I AM NOT OFTEN SICK. I USUALLY TAKE THIS FOR GRANTED, and now and then I remember to feel grateful for the boon. Occasionally I pride myself on it, proud of my distance from those poor fish drying up on the sidewalk. Then I like to push my luck a little—stay up late, skip a meal, run myself a little ragged for the sake of my few remaining years of youth—I like to know what I'm still capable of tolerating, and it's less all the time.

Today I am lying in bed with the first flu I've had in several years. I have a fever, a headache, a tender and queasy stomach—how I hate it. I whine and grumble, sorry for myself. It is as though I've been sick a long, long time. With a vague wistfulness I remember my vigor of just a few days ago, running in the park, bending in the garden, and it seems far away, another woman's strength, out of reach. I padded down to the study yesterday and gathered up my *Merck Manual of Diagnosis and Therapy* and a textbook or two and laid them around me in bed like charms. In alert moments I leaf through the sections on hepatitis, malaria, leukemia. Could this be my turn? Everything seems to start with a "flu-like syndrome." Will the rest of my life be divided into the time before Sunday afternoon, when I went to bed with a fever, and after? What a coward I am; the very idea makes my heart race.

L AST WINTER ONE OF MY TWO CATS CRAWLED UP INTO a car engine, seeking its warmth, and was curled there sleepily when the driver started the engine. Her belly was ripped apart by the fan belt. She stood forlornly by the door, and I picked her up and saw the gaping holes, the muscle wall and torn fat opening to swollen intestines. She survived two infections, two operations, and is still with us—arthritic, a bit strange. Each time she comes home from the vet our other cat bristles—stalks her with tail high, fur up, nose quivering. What is this alien smell, this threat? The sick cat is a pariah, ostracized; once sick, she is outcast for days. In the same way do we bristle and hiss at our weak, embarrassing fellows and their sour, unsavory smells.

A necessary quality of sickness is its casting off of all else, its enforced priority—the way the world pales in its shadow. We can hold it at bay a while by refusing to act the part, but the time comes when we have no choice. If we aren't exactly sick, then neither are we well, and I suspect we never will be. Sickness looks so passive, so inert, and that's part of our contempt: this childishness, this impotence, how those people just *lie there*. This is why we fear death, cannot sanction the act. It seems not an act at all, but the very opposite—paralysis. Fight it, man, we say with the rallying cry of war time, flagged by another course of chemotherapy, a breathing tube, the knife. What is forgotten is the dynamic marshaling of energy that can't be seen. This is the source and the essential meaning of healing: a hidden aggression, cell by cell and thought by thought. It is something that cannot be seen. It is the secret of a peaceful death.

Still, I see Lily, white and bald, retching into her bowl as we talked, used to it. I see Molly's dry, shiny, fragile skin, her taut face, the perpetual blood trickling while she waits. I think of them and still there's that visceral, organic fear. I don't want to be like them. I want to be spared, and sooner or later, I won't be.

How many times have I stood at a bedside watching with satisfaction as the bag hung on the rails fills with watery, pale urine, proof that the diuretic is finally working? I watch with no memory at all, no appreciation for how it must feel to lie there, swollen, draining through a tube in the bladder. I see nothing dynamic, no power. I grieve for my own amnesia. I can lie here and dream of vomiting, of relief, and in a week's time it will be just a dream. I'll stand by the bedside, holding a basin, thinking of something else. The person I watch, a stranger, will roll under the sheets, sweating and chilled, defenseless, calling out in the night for mercy, and I'll slip away.

If we are truly to find a foundation in this play of power and pain, if we are ever to strike a balance in this disproportion, we must first do one thing: embrace death. It is our tradition to do the opposite, of course, to fight and run. Compassion and pain, power and helplessness, health and illness are only life and death. The two together are like two eyes, one bringing depth and perspective to the other.

Our supposed motive is to ease suffering, and out of this great suffering is born. A doctor tells me a long story about a man who came to him very sick, with many medical problems, and spent almost three months in the hospital before he was well enough to be transferred to a nursing home. The patient had such poor veins—stiff, narrow, and small—that his blood had to be withdrawn through his femoral vein, the great throbbing vessel that hides in the hollow between the thigh and the groin. Day after day the needles plunged into that soft space, to gather blood for tests, new tests, old tests, repeat tests. Just before his discharge, the man collapsed and died, and in his inevitable autopsy it was discovered that his femoral vein was filled with an embolus, a clot of blood from all the needles. A portion had broken off and blocked his lung, killing him. When I was told this story I was at least glad that this physician, at least, could see his complicity in the man's fate. But that was not why he told me the story at all. To him it was a parable of the odds physicians struggle against. "His number was up," said the doctor. "That's all. His number was up, after all we'd done for him."

First, do no harm. Every physician, every nurse, is thought to make this vow by the people in his or her hands. Our good intentions are taken for granted. And in order to do no harm, we invent great machines, bloodless and wise, to beat the body into longer life. Now we find ourselves a little lost, watching the sorcerer's broom bringing bucket after bucket of water, threatening at last to drown us in our own efforts. We wonder what to do, and how to know, ever edging away from life—because we turn our backs on death. Health becomes a mere transient grace at the mercy of electronic gods, to be guarded as greedily and jealously as a dog his only bone.

EVEN THE MOST ORDINARY THING IS FREAKISH TO THE man on the table. Those starched whites and shiny steel are so much voodoo to him. If we could only bring ourselves to admit it, if we could remember, we would say it is voodoo to us too. We edge around a circle looking toward the center and not over our shoulders. We shuffle quietly, no cries of joy, no epiphanies—not seeing the sheer size, the massiveness, of all we do not know. We face the center while over our shoulders, out there, are *why* and *how* and *now what*. Out there is the breeze that lifts the hair on the back of one's neck.

Our eye gets finer every day, drawing us down until we are looking at smaller and smaller pieces of the whole. We ride it down, the laser and scope and scanner, until we sit at the side of the cell and try to extrapolate from it the rest of the person. This is one kind of detail, but there are others. By having settled for this one we have made a great relinquishment, a surrender at least as great as the surrender of the sick to their sickness. Brave and sad, they give themselves up to decay and loss; we give ourselves up to the force of the cure. It is as though we were sick, and our machine-driven pride the disease.

What is the name of what we see? We must learn to pay attention to these newfound details. See how the dead man's ring beats a rhythmic click against the autopsy table when the cut is made? I can't brush off the tingle on the back of my neck as I watch. I can't distill the stories I'm hiding away like a pack rat. A note rings in me, far away, as though I, too, lie on the table and feel the knife edge shake me.

DIRECT REFERENCES

p. 8: Elber, Lynn. "Questions Will Follow Transplant." *Oregonian* sunrise ed. (Oct. 28, 1984): A1.

p. 9: Leighty, John M. "Robots Marching into Medical Field." *Oregonian* sunrise ed. (Jan. 24, 1985): D3.

p. 12: Paris, John J. "Terminating Treatment for Newborns: A Theological Perspective." *Law, Medicine, and Health Care* 10, no. 3 (1982): 120–124.

p. 30: Perelman, Robert H., and Farrell, Philip M. "Analysis of Causes of Neonatal Death in the United States with Specific Emphasis on Fatal Hyaline Membrane Disease." *Pediatrics* 70(1982): 570–575.

p. 45: Lozano, Carlos H. "Follow-up Studies of Survivors of Respiratory Distress Syndrome." In *Hyaline Membrane Disease: Pathogenesis and Pathophysiology*, ed. Leo Stern, 273–287. New York: Grune and Stratton, 1984.

p. 45: Bennett, Forrest C., Robinson, Nancy M., and Sells, Clifford J. "Growth and Development of Infants Weighing Less Than 800 Grams at Birth." *Pediatrics* 71(1983)319–323.

p. 47: Krummel, Thomas M., Greenfield, Lazar J., Kirkpatrick, Barry V., Mueller, Dawn G., Kerkering, Kathryn W., and Salzberg, Arnold M. "Extracorporeal Membrane Oxygenation in Neonatal Pulmonary Failure." *Pediatric Annual* 11 (1982):905–908.

p. 49: Paris, John. "Terminating Treatment for Newborns: A Theological Perspective." *Law, Medicine, and Health Care* 10, no. 3(1982):120–124.

p. 49: Committee on the Legal and Ethical Aspects of Health Care for Children. "Comments and Recommendations on the 'Infant Doe' Proposed Regulations." *Law, Medicine and Health Care* 11, no. 5 (1983):203–213.

p. 55: Perlman, Jeffery M., Goodman, Steven, Kreusser, Katherine L., Volpe, Joseph J. "Reduction in Intraventricular Hemorrhage by Elimination of Fluctuating Blood-Flow Velocity in Preterm Infants with Respiratory Distress Syndrome." *New England Journal of Medicine* 312(1985):1353–1357.

p. 63: Whaley, Lucille F., and Wong, Donna L. *Nursing Care of Infants and Children.* St. Louis: C. V. Mosby, 1979.

p. 63: Berkow, Robert, and Talbott, John H. *The Merck Manual of Diagnosis and Therapy* 13th Ed. Rahway, N.J.: Merck, 1977.

p. 64: Kazazian, Haig H. Jr., Leonard, Claire O., and Corson, Virginia. "Prevention of Congenital Malformation Syndromes: Use of New Prenatal Diagnostic Techniques." In *Associated Congenital Anomalies,* ed. M. El Shafie and Charles H. Klippel. Baltimore: Williams & Wilkins, 1981.

p. 64: Ackerman, Terrence F. "Meningomyelocele and Parental Commitment: A Policy Proposal Regarding Selection for Treatment." *Man and Medicine* 5(1980):291–303.

p. 70: Thurow, Lester Carl. "Learning to Say 'No.' " *New England Journal of Medicine* 311(1984):1569–1572.

p. 75: Landsman, Melanie K. "The Patient with Chronic Renal Failure: A Marginal Man." *Annals of Internal Medicine* 82 (1975):268–270.

p. 86: Abram, Harry S. "The 'Uncooperative' Hemodialysis Patient: A Psychiatrist's Viewpoint and a Patient's Commentary." In *Living or Dying,* ed. Norman B. Levy, 50–61. Springfield, Ill.: Charles C. Thomas, 1974.

p. 93: Reichsman, Franz, and Levy, Norman B. "Problems in Adaptation to Maintenance Hemodialysis: A Four-Year Study of 25 Patients." In *Living or Dying.* Op. cit., 30–49.

p. 94: Foster, F. Gordon, Cohn, George L., and McKegney, F. Patrick. "Pyschobiologic Factors and Individual Survival on Chronic Renal Hemodialysis: A Two Year Followup, Part I." In ibid, 74–101.

p. 94: Higgerson, Alicia Beck, and Bulechek, Gloria M. "A Descriptive Study Concerning the Psychosocial Dimensions of Living Related Kidney Donations." *AANNT Journal* 9, no. 6 (1982):27–31.

pp. 98, 102: Abram, Harry S., Kemph, John P., McKegney, F. Patrick, and Scribner, Belding H., with Norman B. Levy, Moderator. "Panel: Living or Dying." In *Living or Dying.* Op. cit., 3–29.

pp. 104, 106: Orr, Martha L. "Cost Containment and Patient Choice in the End Stage Renal Disease Program." *AANNT Journal* 9, no. 6 (1982):11–15.

p. 105: Watson, M. A., Diamandopoulos, A. A., Briggs, J. D., Hamilton, D. N. H., and Dick, H. M. "Endogenous Cell-Mediated Immunity, Blood Transfusion, and Outcome of Renal Transplantation." *The Lancet* (Dec. 22 and 29, 1979): 1323–1326.

p. 106: Reed, Karen. "The Vacaville Inmate Who Wants to Die." *San Francisco Chronicle.* Dec. 26, 1984.

pp. 124, 125: Heidrich, George, Perry, Samuel, and Amand, Robert. "Nursing Staff Attitudes about Burn Pain." *Journal of Burn Care and Rehabilitation* 2(1981):259–261.

p. 125: Torgerson, Warren S. "What Objective Measures Are There for Evaluating Pain?" *The Journal of Trauma* 24, no. 9 (1984):s187–s195.

pp. 126, 127, 143: Kavanaugh, Charlene. "A New Approach to Dressing Change in the Severely Burned Child and Its Effect on Burn-Related Psychopathology." *Heart and Lung* 12(1983):612–618.

pp. 130, 137, 142: Jacoby, Florence Greenhouse. *Nursing Care of the Patient with Burns.* (2d ed.). St. Louis: C. V. Mosby, 1976.

pp. 132, 134, 141, 146: Bernstein, Norman R. *Emotional Care of the Facially Burned and Disfigured.* Boston: Little, Brown, 1976.

p. 138: Imbus, Sharon H., and Zawacki, Bruce E. "Autonomy for Burned Patients When Survival Is Unprecedented." *New England Journal of Medicine* 297(1977):308–310.

p. 139: Frank, Hugh A., and Wachtel, Thomas L. "Life and Death in a Burn Center." *Journal of Burn Care and Rehabilitation* 5(1984):339–341.

p. 140: Nielsen, Judith A., Kolman, Patricia B. R., and Wachtel, Thomas L. "Suicide and Parasuicide by Burning." *Journal of Burn Care and Rehabilitation* 5(1984):335–338.

p. 140: Layton, T. R., and Copeland, C. E. "Burn Suicide." *Journal of Burn Care and Rehabilitation* 4(1983):445–446.

p. 142: Wernick, Robert L., Brantly, Phillip J., and Malcolm, Robert. "Behavioral Techniques in the Psychological Rehabilitation of Burn Patients." *International Journal of Psychiatry in Medicine* 10, no. 2 (1980–81):145–149.

p. 142: West, Donald A., and Shuck, Jerry M. "Emotional Problems of the Severely Burned Patient." *Surgical Clinics of North America* 58(1978):1189–1204.

p. 144: Layton, Thomas R., and Lepore, Shirley A. Letter. *Journal of Burn Care and Rehabilitation* 5(1984):400–401.

p. 175: Luther, Stephen L., Price, James H., and Rose, Cynthia A. "The Public's Knowledge about Cancer." *Cancer Nursing* 5, no. 2 (1982):109–116.

p. 183: Haskell, Charles M. "Drugs Used in Chemotherapy." In *Cancer Treatment,* ed. Charles M. Haskell. Philadelphia: W. B. Saunders, 1985.

p. 189: Batzdorf, Ulrich, and Catlin, Don H. "Pain Syndromes in Malignant

Disease." In *Cancer Treatment*, ed. Charles M. Haskell. Philadelphia: W. B. Saunders, 1985.

p. 189: Rankin, Margaret A. "Use of Drugs for Pain with Cancer Patients." *Cancer Nursing* 5, no. 2 (1982):181–190.

p. 189: Anderson, Jamie Lavenia. "Nursing Management of the Cancer Patient in Pain: A Review of the Literature by Jamie Lavenia Anderson." *Cancer Nursing* 5, no. 1 (1982):33–41.

p. 190: Degner, Wesley F., Fujii, Samuel H., and Levitt, Martin. "Implementing a Program to Control Chronic Pain of Malignant Disease for Patients in an Extended Care Facility." *Cancer Nursing* 5, no. 4 (1982):263–268.

p. 190: Marks, Richard M., and Sachar, Edward J. "Undertreatment of Medical Inpatients with Narcotic Analgesics." *Annals of Internal Medicine* 78-(1973):173–181.

p. 190: Rankin, Margaret A., and Snider, Bill. "Nurses' Perceptions of Cancer Patients' Pain." *Cancer Nursing* 7, no. 2 (1984):149–155.

p. 204: Oye, Robert K., Shapiro, Martin F., "Reporting Results from Chemotherapy Trials: Does Response Make a Difference in Patient Survival?" *Journal of American Medical Association* 252(1984):2722–2725.

p. 204: Becker, Teresa M. *Basics of Cancer Chemotherapy.* Boston: Little, Brown, 1981.

p. 206: Moertal, Charles G., Fleming, Thomas R., Creagan, Edward T., Rubin, Joseph, O'Connell, Michael J., and Ames, Matthew M. "High-Dose Vitamin C versus Placebo in the Treatment of Patients with Advanced Cancer Who Have Had No Prior Chemotherapy." *New England Journal of Medicine* 312(1985)137–141.

p. 208: Lee, Helen J. "Analysis of a Concept: Hardiness." *Oncology Nursing Forum* 10, no. 4 (1983):32–35.

pp. 232, 234: Smith, Orville. "Primates in Biomedical Study: Resources to be Conserved." *Research Resources Reporter* December (1982): 1–3.

p. 235: Wiesenfeld-Hallin, Z. "The Effects of Intrathecal Morphine and Naltrexone on Autotomy in Sciatic Nerve Sectioned Rats." *Pain* 18(1984):267–278.

p. 236: Wellisch, David K., and Cohen, Robin S. "Psychosocial Aspects of Cancer." In *Cancer Treatment*, ed. Charles M. Haskell. Philadelphia: W. B. Saunders, 1985.

p. 237: Mistretta, Charlotte M., and Bradley, Robert M. "Taste in Utero: Theoretical Considerations." In *Taste and Development: The Genesis of Sweet Preference*, James M. Weiffenbach, 51–63. National Institute of Dental Research, 1977.

BACKGROUND
REFERENCES

(alphabetical)

American Cancer Society. *A Guide to Services and Information for Cancer Patients in the Portland Metropolitan Area.* Portland, Oreg.: American Cancer Society, 1984.

Averette, Hervy E., and Sevin, Bernd-Uloe. "Debulking Surgery and Second Look Operation." *International Journal of Radiation, Oncology, Biology, and Physics* 8(1981):891–892.

Bach, F. H. "Immunogenetics of Tissue Grafting." In *The Treatment of Renal Failure,* ed. J. E. Castro, 313–322. New York: Appleton-Century Crofts, 1982.

Bauers, Christina M. "A Review of the End-Stage Renal Disease Program." *Nephrology Nurse* 5, no. 4 (1983):17–22.

Beattie, Edward J., and Cowan, Stuart D. *Toward the Conquest of Cancer.* New York: Crown, 1980.

Berek, Jonathan S., Hacker, Neville F., and Lagasse, Leo D. "Ovarian Cancer." In *Cancer Treatment,* ed. Charles M. Haskell. Philadelphia: W. B. Saunders, 1985.

Bowd, Alan D. "Ethical Reservations about Psychological Research with Animals." *The Psychological Record* 30(1980):201–210.

Cahill, Kevin M., ed. *The AIDS Epidemic.* New York: St. Martin's Press, 1983.

Calne, R. Y., Thiru, S., McMaster, P., Craddock, G. N., White, D. J. G., Evans, D. B., Dunn, D. C., Pentlow, B. D., and Rolles, Keith. "Cyclosporin A in Patients Receiving Renal Allografts from Cadaver Donors." *The Lancet* (December 23 and 30, 1978): 1323–1327.

Calne, R. Y. "Transplant Surgery: Current Status." *British Journal of Surgery* 67(1980):765–771.

Cason, J. S. *Treatment of Burns.* London: Chapman and Hall, 1981.

Castro, J. E., ed. *The Treatment of Renal Failure*, 323–379. New York: Appleton-Century Crofts, 1982.

Chang, Frederic C., and Herzog, Briant. "Burn Morbidity: A Follow-up Study of Physical and Psychological Disability." *Annals of Surgery* 183(1976):34–37.

Clarke, A. Murray, and Martin, H. L. "The Effects of Previous Thermal Injury on Adolescents." *Burns* 5, no. 1 (1978):101–104.

Consensus Conference. "Total Hip-Joint Replacement in the United States." *Journal of the American Medical Association* 248(1982):1817–1821.

Curtin, Leah. "Should We Feed Baby Doe?" *Nursing Management* 15, no. 8 (1984):22–28.

Davis, Faye D. "Current Strategies in the Procurement of Cadaveric Kidneys for Transplantation." *Nursing Clinics of North America* 16(1981):565–571.

"Defibrillator Recall Ordered." *The Oregonian* sunrise ed. (Mar. 16, 1985):B5.

Deitch, E. A., and Staats, M. "Child Abuse through Burning." *Journal of Burn Care and Rehabilitation* 3(1982):89–94.

Faccini, E., Uzumaki, H., Govoni, S., Missale, C., Spano, P. F., Covelli, V., and Trabucchi, M. "Afferent Fibers Mediate the Increase of Met-Enkephalin Elicited in Rat Spinal Cord by Localized Pain." *Pain* 18(1984):25–31.

Fettner, Ann Giudici, and Check, William A. *The Truth about AIDS: Evolution of an Epidemic.* New York: Holt, Rinehart & Winston, 1984.

Fidler, James P. "Debridement and Grafting of Full-Thickness Burns." *Clinical Burn Therapy: A Management and Prevention Guide*, ed. Robert P. Hummel, 111–138. Boston: PSG Inc., 1982.

Flynn, John T. "Oxygen and Retrolental Fibroplasia: Update and Challenge." *Journal of Anesthesiology* 60(1984):397–399.

Frey, R. G. "Vivisection, Morals, and Medicine." *Journal of Medical Ethics* 9(1983):94–97.

Frey, R. G. "Response." *Journal of Medical Ethics* 9(1983):104.

Fuk, Zvi, Rizel, Shulamit, Anteby, Shaoul O., and Biran, Shoshana. "The Multimodal Approach to the Treatment of Stage III Ovarian Carcinoma." *International Journal of Radiation, Oncology, Biology, and Physics* 8(1981):903–908.

Glass, Penny, Avery, Gorden B., Subramanian, Kolinjavadi N. Siva, Keys, Marshall P., Soster, Anita M., and Friendly, David S. "Effect of Bright Light in the Hospital Nursery on the Incidence of Retinopathy of Prematurity." *New England Journal of Medicine* 313(1985):401–404.

Goldsmith, Charles E. "Illness Behavior of Dialysis Patients, Staff Response, and Coping Measures." *AANNT Journal* 9, no. 6 (1982):38–41.

Greene, Jamie G., Fox, Nathan A., Lewis, Michael. "The Relationship between Neonatal Characteristics and Three-Month Mother-Infant Interaction in High-Risk Infants." *Child Development* 54(1983):1286–1296.

Haskell, Charles M. In *Cancer Treatment*. Philadelphia: W. B. Saunders, 1985.

Haskell, Charles M., Guiliano, Armando E., Thompson, Ronald W., Zarem, Harvey A. "Breast Cancer." In *Cancer Treatment*, ed. Charles M. Haskell. Philadelphia: W. B. Saunders, 1985.

Higginson, John. "The Face of Cancer Worldwide." *Hospital Practice* November (1983):145–157.

Hodson, W. Alan and Truog, William E. *Critical Care of the Newborn*. Philadelphia: W. B. Saunders, 1983.

Johnson, Carole L., O'Shaughnessy, Edward J., Ostergren, Gregg. *Burn Management*. New York: Raven Press, 1981.

Johnson, John W. C., Beck, Jeanne C., Haberkern, Charles M. "Glucocorticoids and the Respiratory Distress Syndrome." In *Obstetrics and Gynecology Annual*, ed. Ralph M. Wynn, 99–130. New York: Appleton-Century Crofts, 1984.

Kennedy, C. R. "Ovarian Cancer: The Ten-Year Experience of a District General Hospital." *British Journal of Obstetrics and Gynecology* 88-(1981):1186–1191.

Kennedy, Donald. "Remarks to the California Biomedical Research Association." Palo Alto, Calif.: Stanford University, April 30, 1984.

Kerstern, Robert C., and Kolder, Hansjoerg E. "Intraocular Lens Implantation: Residents vs. Staff." *Ophthalmic Surgery* 13(1982):470–472.

Klahr, Saulo, Nolph, Karl D., and Luke, Robert G. *End-Stage Renal Disease: Pathophysiology, Dialysis, and Transplantation*. Rockville, Md.: National Center for Health Care Technology, Dept. of Health and Human Services, 1981.

Klaus, Marshall H. and Fanaroll, Avroy A. (Ed.) *Care of the High-Risk Neonate*, 2nd Ed. Philadelphia: W. B. Saunders, 1979.

Kolman, Patricia B. R. "The Incidence of Psychopathology in Burned Adult Patients: A Critical Review." *Journal of Burn Care and Rehabilitation* 4(1983):430–436.

Law, Edward J. "Minimizing Burn Scar and Contracture." *Clinical Burn Therapy: A Management and Prevention Guide*, ed. Robert P. Hummel, 301–320. Boston: PSG Inc., 1982.

Lorber, John. "Incidence and Epidemiology of Myelomeningocele." *Clinical Orthopedics and Related Research* 45(1966):81–83.

Lyon, Jeff. *Playing God in the Nursery*. New York: W. W. Norton, 1985.

Medical Research Council's Working Party on Ovarian Cancer, "Medical Research Council Study on Chemotherapy in Advanced Ovarian Cancer." *British Journal of Obstetrics and Gynaecology* 88(1981):1174–1185.

Miyake, Kensaku, Asakura, Masako, and Kobayashi, Hiroko. "Effect of Intraocular Lens Fixation on the Blood-Aqueous Barrier." *American Journal of Ophthamology* 98(1984):451–455.

Molnar, G. E., and Taft, L. T. "Pediatric Rehabilitation Part II: Spina Bifida and Limb Deficiencies." *Current Problems in Pediatrics* 7, no. 4 (1977):3–31.

Morris, Peter J. "Histocompatibility Antigens in Human Organ Transplants." *Surgical Clinics of North America*. 58(1978):233–244.

National Academy of Sciences. *Animals for Research: A Directory of Sources*. (10th ed.) Institute of Laboratory Animal Resources, National Research Council, National Academy of Sciences, 1979.

Nevitt, Michael C., Epstein, Wallace V., Masem, Mathias, and Murray, William R. "Work Disability before and after Total Hip Arthroplasty." *Arthritis and Rheumatism* 27(1984):410–420.

Palmer, John M., and Chatterjee, Satya N. "Urologic Complications in Renal Transplants." *Surgical Clinics of North America*. 58(1978):305–320.

Perry, Samuel, and Black, Karen. "Delirium in Burn Patients." *Journal of Burn Care and Rehabilitation* 5(1984):210–214.

Regan, Tom. *The Case for Animal Rights*. Berkeley, Calif.: University of California Press, 1984.

Rodriguez, Donna J., and Hunter, Virginia M. "Nutritional Intervention in the Treatment of Chronic Renal Failure." *Nursing Clinics of North America* 16(1981):573–578.

Rosenberg, Steven A. "The Impact of Emerging Biotechnology on Cancer Care." *American College of Surgeons Bulletin* 69, no. 9 (1984):2.

Sheldon, Roger E., and Dominiak, Pat Sellars, Ed. *The Expanding Role of the Nurse in Neonatal Intensive Care*. New York: Grune and Stratton, 1980.

Sievers, Hermine, and von Domarus, Dietrich. "Foreign-Body Reaction

Against Intraocular Lenses." *American Journal of Ophthamology* 97(1984):743–751.

Singer, Peter. *Animal Liberation*. New York: Avon, 1975.

Sprigge, T. L. S. "Vivisection, morals, medicine: commentary from an antivivisectionist philosopher." *Journal of Medical Ethics* 9(1983):98–101.

Stark, June L., and Hunt, Valerie. "Helping Your Patient with Chronic Renal Failure." *Nursing* 13, no. 9 (1983):56–63.

Stark, Walter J., Leske, Cristina M., Worthen, David M., and Murray, George C. "Trends in Cataract Surgery and Intraocular Lenses in the United States." *American Journal of Ophthalmology* 96(1984):743–751.

Stark, Walter J., Terry, Arlo C., Worthen, David, and Murray, George C. "Update of Intraocular Lenses Implanted in the United States." *American Journal of Ophthalmology* 98 (1984):238–239.

Taub, Sheila. "Cancer and the Law of Informed Consent." *Law, Medicine, and Health Care* April (1982):61–90.

Taub, Sheila. "Withholding Treatment from Defective Newborns." *Law, Medicine and Health Care* 10, no. 1 (1982):4–10.

Thoft, Richard A. "The Role of Lens Implantation in Cataract Surgery." *Annual Review of Medicine* 35(1984):595–604.

U.S. Dept. of Health and Human Services. *Medicare Annual Report: Fiscal Year 1981*. GPO, 1983.

U.S. Dept. of Health and Human Services. *Taking Time: Support For People With Cancer and the People Who Care About Them*. Bethesda, Md: National Cancer Institute, 1983.

U.S. Health Care Financing Administration. *End-Stage Renal Disease Program Highlights*. GPO, 1984.

Walkenstein, Merri D. "Comparison of Burned Patients' Perception of Pain With Nurses' Perception of Patients' Pain." *Journal of Burn Care and Rehabilitation* 3(1982):233–236.

Williams, G. Melville. "Status of Renal Transplantation Today." *Surgical Clinics of North America* 58(1978):273–285.

Woodward, Joan. "Emotional Disturbances of Burned Children." *British Medical Journal* (1959):1009–1013.

Young, Robert C., Myers, Charles E., Ozols, Robert F., and Hogan, W. Michael. "Chemotherapy in Advanced Disease." *International Journal of Radiation, Oncology, Biology, and Physics* 8(1981):889–902.

Zak, Thaddeus A. "Retinopathy of Prematurity." *New York State Journal of Medicine* 82(1982):1795–1796.

Index